"The Wordsworth of healing."
 –Ella Boyce Kirk, author of *My Pilgrimage to Coué*

"You will love this unique man – unique by reason of his noble charity and his unselfish love of his brethren as Christ has taught it. And like myself, you will be healed physically, morally and mentally. Life will seem more worth living and altogether more beautiful. And that is surely worth trying for."
 –Marguerite Burnat-Provins, author of *Le Livre Pour Toi*

"He succeeds in a simple way of stripping disease of its dignity."
 –George Draper, *Literary Digest*

"The more one listens to Mr. Coué, the more one likes him, and the more his theories and methods exchange mystery for simplicity."
 –Robert Littell, *New Republic*

"If every teacher had Mr. Coué's kindliness, charm, shrewdness, and simplicity, young people would go to school and college for the fun that they could get in their classrooms as well as on their playing fields."
 –Ernest Hamlin Abbott, *The Outlook*

"A man whose devotion is rivaled by his modesty."
 –Charles Baudouin, author of *Suggestion and Autosuggestion*

# SIMPLE SELF-HEALING
## THE MAGIC OF AUTOSUGGESTION

TAUGHT BY
### *ÉMILE COUÉ*

WITH ADDITIONAL COMMENTARY BY
### *CYRUS HARRY BROOKS*

EDITED AND ADAPTED BY
### *TIM GRIMES*

**RADICAL COUNSELOR**
**CAMBRIDGE, MASSACHUSETTS**

FOR MORE INFORMATION VISIT:

## *www.radicalcounselor.com*

PUBLISHED BY TIM GRIMES, CAMBRIDGE MA

*Simple Self-Healing: The Magic of Autosuggestion*
Copyright © 2017 by Tim Grimes

This book was adapted from:
*Self-Mastery Through Conscious Autosuggestion*
by Émile Coué, originally published in 1922
*The Practice of Autosuggestion*
by Cyrus Harry Brooks, originally published in 1922
*My Method: Including American Impressions*
by Émile Coué, originally published in 1923

LIBRARY OF CONGRESS CONTROL NUMBER: 2017939412
ISBN-13: 978-1545232729
ISBN-10: 1545232725
PRINTED IN THE UNITED STATES OF AMERICA

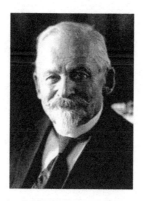

ÉMILE COUÉ
(1857-1926)

*"Repeat twenty times, morning and evening: 'Every day, in every way, I'm getting better and better.' It's the same remedy for everybody in the world. It's so simple and so easy. Almost too easy, isn't it? But this is important: If you have the thought in your mind that you're sick, you surely will be. If you think you're going to be cured, it's sure to happen. It's the certainty that you're about to recover that brings results, not the hope."*

# CONTENTS

## Editor's Note

French psychologist Émile Coué was one of the more underappreciated geniuses of 20th century medicine. Almost a hundred years ago, Coué's popular self-healing method – which he called autosuggestion – helped cure thousands of people annually. Today, however, few people have ever even heard of Coué. Once considered to be on par with the discoveries of Freud, autosuggestion faded into the background upon Coué's death, and has largely been forgotten. This book will introduce you to Coué's overlooked formula – while surprising you in the process.

The practical healing method you're about to learn about is simple. It may seem *too* simple: We don't like solutions to appear this obvious. Autosuggestion's neglect is an example of such a paradox. We often prefer complicated solutions over simpler ones – even when the simple answers can work just as well, or even better. So repeating a short phrase to help solve a problem – like *"Every day, in every way, I'm getting better and better"* – initially seems ridiculous to most of us. But it's not. And this book will reveal to you why.

*Simple Self-Healing* begins with Cyrus Harry Brooks' vivid introduction of Coué at work, and then is followed by recommendations Coué made after teaching autosuggestion in the United States. Coué's advice is divided into short chapters, for ease and clarity, as he makes points that are highly perceptive, and worth repeated referral. The book also includes additional insights by Brooks on Coué's method, as well as various quotes attributed to Coué (originally recorded by Émile Léon) and examples of Coué teaching autosuggestion to others.

The overall scope of *Simple Self-Healing* will make you understand how easy and practical autosuggestion is to apply, even in modern times. The information has been adapted to provide you with clarity on this neglected subject. If you grasp the simplicity of autosuggestion, you'll be able to use this wonderful tool as you wish – and it should help make your life "better and better." Enjoy.

*–Tim Grimes*

# A Quick Summary of
# the General Formula

Every morning upon waking, and every evening as soon as you're in bed, close your eyes. Without fixing your attention on what you say, pronounce about twenty times – just loud enough so you can hear your own words – the following phrase:

*"Every day, in every way, I'm getting better and better."*

The words "in every way" are good for anything and everything – it's not necessary to formulate particular autosuggestions.

Repeat this phrase with faith and confidence, and with the certainty that you're going to obtain what you desire.

Moreover, if during the day or night you have a physical or mental pain, or feel depressed, immediately affirm to yourself that you're not going to consciously contribute anything to maintain that pain or depression – but that it will disappear quickly. Then isolate yourself as much as possible. Close your eyes, and pass your hand across your forehead if your trouble is mental – or over the aching part of your body if your trouble is physical – and repeat quickly, moving your lips, the words:

*"It passes, it passes, it passes…"*

Continue repeating this as long as may be necessary, until the mental or physical pain has disappeared – which it usually does within twenty or twenty-five seconds. Begin again every time you find it necessary to do so. Like the first autosuggestion given above, you must repeat this one also with absolute faith and confidence – but calmly, without effort. Repeat the formula as litanies are repeated in church.

*–Émile Coué*

# INTRODUCTION

*BY CYRUS HARRY BROOKS*

*"Repeat often what you desire – for instance, 'I'm gaining poise,' and you will; 'My memory improves,' and it certainly will improve; 'I'm able to control myself absolutely,' and there's no question that you will."*

## THE CLINIC OF ÉMILE COUÉ

The clinic of Émile Coué, where induced autosuggestion is applied to the treatment of disease, is situated in a pleasant garden attached to his house at the quiet end of the rue Jeanne d'Arc in Nancy. It was here that I visited him in the early summer of 1921, and had the pleasure for the first time of witnessing one of his consultations.

We entered the garden from his house a little before nine o'clock. In one corner was a brick building of two stories with its windows thrown wide open to let in the air and sunshine — this was the clinic. A few yards away was a smaller one-storied construction which served as a waiting room. Under the plum and cherry trees, now laden with fruit, little groups of patients were sitting on the garden seats, chatting amicably together and enjoying the morning sunshine, while others wandered in twos and threes among the flowers and strawberry beds.

The room reserved for the treatments was already crowded, but in spite of that, eager newcomers constantly tried to gain entrance. The windowsills on the ground floor were sat upon, and a dense knot of people had formed in the doorway. Inside, the patients had first occupied the seats which surrounded the walls, and then covered the available floor-space, sitting on campstools and folding-chairs. Coué, with some difficulty, found me a seat, and the treatments immediately began.

The first patient he addressed was a frail, middle-aged man who – accompanied by his daughter – had just arrived from Paris to meet him. The man was a bad case of nervous trouble. He walked with difficulty, and his head, arms and legs were afflicted with a continual tremor. He explained that if he encountered a stranger when walking in the street, the idea that the latter would remark on his infirmity completely paralyzed him, and he had to cling to whatever support was at hand to save himself from falling.

At Coué's invitation, he rose from his seat and took a few steps across the floor. He walked slowly, leaning on a stick; his knees were half bent, and his feet dragged heavily along the ground. Coué encouraged him with the promise of improvement: "You've been sowing bad seed in your unconscious; now you will sow good seed. The power by which you have produced these ill effects will in future produce equally good ones."

The next patient was an excitable, overworked woman of the artisan class. When Coué inquired about the nature of her trouble, she broke into a flood of complaints, describing each symptom with a voluble exactness. "Madame," he interrupted, "you think too much about your ailments, and in thinking of them you create fresh ones."

Next came a girl with headaches, a youth with

inflamed eyes, and a farm-laborer incapacitated by varicose veins. In each case, Coué stated that autosuggestion should bring complete relief. Then it was the turn of a businessman who complained of nervousness, lack of self-confidence and haunting fears.

"When you know the method," said Coué, "You'll not allow yourself to harbor such ideas."

"I work terribly hard to get rid of them," the patient answered.

"You fatigue yourself. The greater effort you make, the more the ideas return. You'll change all that easily, simply, and above all – without effort."

"I want to," the man interjected.

"That's just where you're wrong," Coué told him. "If you say 'I want to do something,' your imagination replies 'Oh, but you can't.' You must say *'I am going to do it,'* and if it's in the region of the possible, you'll succeed."

A little further on was another neurasthenic — a girl. This was her third visit to the clinic, and for ten days she'd been practicing the method at home. With a happy smile, and a little pardonable self-importance, she declared that she already felt a considerable improvement. She had more energy, was beginning to enjoy life, ate heartily and slept more soundly. Her sincerity and naive delight helped to strengthen the faith of her fellow patients. They looked on her as a living proof of the healing which should come to themselves.

Coué continued his questions. Those who were unable,

whether through rheumatism or some paralytic affection, to make use of a limb were called on – as a criterion of future progress – to put out their maximum efforts.

In addition, there were present a man and a woman who could not walk without support, and a burly peasant, formerly a blacksmith, who for nearly ten years had not succeeded in lifting his right arm above the level of his shoulder. In each case, Coué predicted a complete cure.

During this preliminary stage of the treatment, the words he spoke were not in the nature of suggestions. They were sober expressions of opinion, based on years of experience. Not once did he reject the possibility of cure, though with several patients suffering from organic disease in an advanced stage, he admitted its unlikelihood. To these he promised, however, a cessation of pain, an improvement of morale, and at least a retardment of the progress of the disease.

"Meanwhile," he added, "the limits of the power of autosuggestion aren't yet known; final recovery is possible." In all cases of functional and nervous disorders – as well as the less serious ones of an organic nature – he stated that autosuggestion, conscientiously applied, was capable of removing the trouble completely.

It took Coué nearly forty minutes to complete his interrogation. Other patients bore witness to the benefits the treatment had already conferred on them. A woman with a painful swelling in her breast, which a doctor had diagnosed (in Coué's opinion, wrongly) as of a cancerous nature, had found complete relief after less than three weeks' treatment. Another woman had enriched her impoverished blood, and increased her weight by over nine pounds. A man had been cured of a varicose ulcer; another in a single sitting had rid himself of a lifelong habit of stammering. Only one of the former patients failed to report an improvement.

"Monsieur," said Coué to him, "You've been making efforts. You must put your trust in the imagination, not in the will. Think you are better, and you will become so." Coué then proceeded to outline the theory given in the pages which follow. It's sufficient here to state his main conclusions, which were these:

1. *Every idea which exclusively occupies the mind is transformed into an actual physical or mental state.*

2. *The efforts we make to conquer an idea by exerting willpower only serve to make that idea more powerful.*

To demonstrate these truths, he requested one of his patients – a young, anemic-looking woman – to carry out a small experiment. She extended her arms in front of her, and clasped her hands firmly together with the fingers interlaced, increasing the force of her grip until a slight tremor set in. "Look at your hands," said Coué, "and think you would like to open them, *but you cannot*...Now try and pull them apart. Pull hard. You find that the more you try, the more tightly they become clasped together."

The girl made little convulsive movements of her wrists, really doing her best by physical force to separate her hands – but the harder she tried, the more her grip increased in strength, until the knuckles turned white with the pressure. Her hands seemed locked together by a force outside her own control.

"Now think," said Coué, " '*I can open my hands.* '"

Slowly, her grasp relaxed and – in response to a little pull – the cramped fingers came apart. She smiled shyly at the attention she had attracted, and sat down. Coué pointed out that the two main points of his theory were just demonstrated simultaneously: When the patient's mind was filled with the thought *"I cannot,"* she couldn't in fact unclasp her hands. Furthermore, the efforts she made to wrench them apart by exerting her will only fixed them more firmly together.

Each patient was now called on in turn to perform the same experiment. The more imaginative among them — notably the women — were at once successful. One old lady was so absorbed in the thought "I cannot" as not to heed the request to think "I can." With her face ruefully puckered up she sat staring fixedly at her interlocked fingers, as though contemplating an act of fate. "Voilà," said Coué smiling, "if Madame persists in her present idea, she'll never open her hands again as long as she lives."

Several of the men, however, were not at once successful. The former blacksmith with the disabled arm, when told to think "I should like to open my hands but I cannot," proceeded without difficulty to open them.

"You see," said Coué, with a smile, "it depends not on what I say but on what you think. What were you thinking then?"

He hesitated. "I thought perhaps I could open them after all."

"Exactly. And therefore, you could. Now clasp your hands again. Press them together."

When the right degree of pressure had been reached, Coué told him to repeat the words *"I can't, I can't, I can't..."*

As he repeated this phrase the contraction increased, and all his efforts failed to release his grip.

"Voilà," said Coué. "Now listen. For ten years you've been thinking you couldn't lift your arm above your shoulder. Consequently, you haven't been able to do so, for whatever we think becomes true for us. Now think *'I can lift it.'*"

The patient looked at him doubtfully.

"Quick!" Coué said in a tone of authority. "Think *'I can, I can!'*"

"I can," said the man. He made a half-hearted attempt and complained of a pain in his shoulder.

"Bon," said Coué. "Don't lower your arm. Close your eyes and repeat with me as fast as you can: *'Ça passe, ça passe, ça passe...'*"

For half a minute, they repeated this phrase together, speaking so fast as to produce a sound like the whirr of a rapidly revolving machine. Meanwhile Coué quickly stroked the man's shoulder. At the end of that time the patient admitted that his pain had left him.

"Now think that you can lift your arm," Coué said.

The departure of the pain had given the patient faith. His face, which before had been perplexed and incredulous, brightened as the thought of power took possession of him.

"I can," he said in a tone of finality, and without effort he calmly lifted his arm to its full height above his head. He held it there triumphantly for a moment while the whole company applauded and encouraged him.

Coué reached for his hand and shook it.

"My friend, you're cured."

"C'est merveilleux," the man answered. "I believe I am."

"Prove it," said Coué. "Hit me on the shoulder."

The patient laughed, and dealt him a gentle rap.

"Harder," Coué encouraged him. "Hit me harder – as hard as you can."

His arm began to rise and fall in regular blows, increasing in force until Coué was compelled to call on him to stop.

"Voilà, mon ami, you can go back to your anvil."

The man resumed his seat, still hardly able to comprehend what had occurred. Now and then he lifted his arm as if to reassure himself, whispering to himself in an awed voice, "I can, I can."

A little further on was seated a woman who had complained of violent neuralgia. Under the influence of the repeated phrase *"ça passe"* (it passes) the pain was dispelled in less than thirty seconds. Then it was the turn of the visitor from Paris. What he had seen had inspired him with confidence: He was sitting more erect, there was a little patch of color in his cheeks, and his trembling seemed less violent.

He performed the experiment with immediate success.

"Now," said Coué, "you're cultivated ground. I can throw out the seed in handfuls."

He had the sufferer first stand erect with his back and knees straightened. Then he instructed him, while constantly thinking *"I can,"* to place his entire weight on each foot in turn, slowly performing the military exercise known as "marking time." A space was then cleared of chairs, and having discarded his stick, the man was made to walk to and fro. When his gait became slovenly Coué stopped him, pointed out his fault, and, renewing the thought *"I can,"* caused him to correct it.

Progressive improvement kindled the man's imagination. He took himself in his own hands. His bearing became more and more confident, he walked more easily, more quickly. His little daughter, all smiles and happy self-forgetfulness, stood beside him uttering expressions of delight, admiration and encouragement. The whole company laughed and clapped their hands.

"After the sitting," said Coué, "you shall come for a run in my garden."

Thus Coué continued his round of the clinic. Each patient suffering from pain was given complete or partial relief; those with useless limbs had a varying measure of use restored to them. Coué's manner was always quietly inspiring. There was no formality, no attitude of the superior person – he treated everyone, whether rich or poor, with the same friendly solicitude.

But, within these limits, he varied his tone to suit the temperament of the patient. Sometimes he was firm, sometimes gently bantering. He seized every opportunity for a little humorous by-play. One might almost say that he tactfully teased some of his patients, giving them an idea that their ailment was absurd, and a little unworthy – that to be ill was a quaint but reprehensible weakness, which they should quickly get rid of.

Indeed, this denial of the dignity of disease is one of the characteristics of the place. No homage is paid to it as a Dread Monarch. It's gently ridiculed, its terrors are made to appear second-rate, and its victims end by laughing at it.

Coué now passed on to the formulation of specific suggestions. The patients closed their eyes and he proceeded in a low, monotonous voice to evoke in their minds the states of health – mental and physical – they were seeking. As they listened to him, their alertness ebbed away; they were lulled into a drowsy state, filled only by the vivid images he called up before the eyes of the mind. The faint rustle of the trees, the songs of the birds, the low voices of those waiting in the garden, merged into a pleasant background, on which his words stood out powerfully. This is what he said:

"Say to yourself that all the words I'm about to utter will be fixed, imprinted and engraved in your minds. That they'll remain fixed, imprinted and engraved there, so that without your will and knowledge, without your being in any way aware of what is taking place, you yourself and your whole organism will obey them...

"I tell you first that every day, three times a day – morning, noon and evening – at mealtime, you'll be hungry. That's to say you'll feel that pleasant sensation which makes us think and say, 'I'd like something to eat!' You'll then eat with excellent appetite, enjoying your food, but you'll never eat too much. You'll eat the right amount, neither too much nor too little, and you'll know intuitively when you've had a sufficient amount. You'll masticate your food thoroughly, transforming it into a smooth paste before swallowing it. In these conditions, you'll digest it well and feel no discomfort of any kind either in the stomach or the intestines. Assimilation will be perfectly performed, and your organism will make the best possible use of the food to create blood, muscle, strength, energy – in a word: *Life*.

"Since you've digested your food properly, the excretory functions will be normally performed. This will take place every morning immediately on rising, and without you having need of any laxative medicine or artificial means of any kind.

"Every night you'll fall asleep at the hour you wish, and will continue to sleep until the hour at which you desire to wake next morning. Your sleep will be calm, peaceful and profound, untroubled by bad dreams or undesirable states of body. You may dream, but your dreams will be pleasant ones. On waking you'll feel well, bright, alert and eager for the day's tasks.

"If in the past, you've been subject to depression, gloom and melancholy forebodings, you'll from now on be free from such troubles. Instead of being moody, anxious and depressed, you'll be cheerful and happy. You'll be happy even if you have no particular reason for being so, just as in the past you were – without good reason – unhappy. I tell you even that if you have serious cause to be worried or depressed, you'll not be so.

"If you've been impatient or ill-tempered, you'll no longer be anything of the kind – on the contrary, you'll always be patient and self-controlled. The happenings which used to irritate you will leave you entirely calm and unmoved.

"If you've sometimes been haunted by evil and unwholesome ideas, by fears or phobias, these ideas will gradually cease to occupy your mind. They'll melt away like a cloud. As a dream vanishes when we wake, so will these vain images disappear.

"I add that all your organs do their work perfectly. Your heart beats normally and the circulation of the blood takes place as it should. The lungs do their work well. The stomach, the intestines, the liver, the biliary duct, the kidneys and the bladder – all carry out their functions correctly. If at present any of the organs named is out of order, the disturbance will grow less day by day, so that within a short space of time it'll have entirely disappeared, and the organ will have resumed its normal function.

"Further, if any organ has a structural lesion, it will from this day be gradually repaired, and in a short period will be completely restored. This will be so even if you're unaware that the trouble exists.

"I must also add – and it's extremely important – that if in the past you've lacked confidence in yourself, this self-distrust will gradually disappear. You'll have confidence in yourself. I repeat: *You will have confidence*.

"Your confidence will be based on the knowledge of the immense power which is within you, by which you can accomplish any task of which your reason approves. With this confidence, you'll be able to do anything you wish to do, provided it's reasonable, and anything that it's your duty to do.

"When you have any task to perform, you'll always think that it's easy. Such words as 'difficult,' 'impossible' and 'I can't' will disappear from your vocabulary. Their place will be taken by this phrase: *'It's easy and I can.'*

"So, considering your work easy – even if it's difficult to others – it'll become easy to you. You'll do it easily, without effort and without fatigue."

These general suggestions were succeeded by particular suggestions referring to the special ailments from which Coué's patients were suffering. Taking each case in turn, he allowed his hand to rest lightly on the heads of the sufferers, while picturing to their minds the health and vigor with which they would soon be endowed. To a woman with an ulcerated leg he spoke as follows: "From now on, your body will do all that's necessary to restore your leg to perfect health. It'll rapidly heal: The tissues will regain their tone; the skin will be soft and healthy. In a short space of time your leg will be vigorous and strong, and will always remain so in the future."

Each special complaint was thus treated with a few appropriate phrases. When he had finished, and the patients were called on to open their eyes, a faint sigh went around the room, as if they were awaking reluctantly from a delicious dream.

Coué now explained to his patients that he possessed no healing powers, and had never healed a person in his life: They carried in themselves the instrument of their own well-being. The results they'd seen were due to the realization of each patient's own thought. He had been merely an agent calling the ideas of health into their minds. Henceforth, they could – and must – be the pilots of their own destiny. He then requested them to repeat, under conditions which will be later defined, the phrase with which his name is associated: *"Every day, in every way, I'm getting better and better."*

The sitting was at an end. The patients rose and crowded around Coué, asking questions, thanking him, shaking him by the hand. Some declared they were already cured, some that they were much better, others that they were confident of cure in the future. It was as if a burden of depression had fallen from their minds. Those who had entered with minds crushed and oppressed went out with hope and optimism shining in their faces.

But Coué waved aside these too insistent admirers, and

beckoning to the three patients who couldn't walk, led them to a corner of the garden where there was a stretch of gravel path running beneath the boughs of fruit trees. Once more impressing on their minds the thought of strength and power, he induced each one to walk without support down this path.

He then invited them to run. They hesitated, but he insisted, telling them that they could run, that they ought to run, that they had but to believe in their own power, and their thought would be manifested in action. They started rather uncertainly, but Coué followed them with persistent encouragements. They began to raise their heads, to lift their feet from the ground and run with greater freedom and confidence. Turning at the end of the path they came back at a fair pace. Their movements weren't elegant, but people on the other side of fifty are rarely elegant runners.

It was a surprising sight to see these three sufferers – who had hobbled to the clinic on sticks – now covering the ground at a full five miles an hour, and laughing heartily at themselves as they ran. The crowd of patients who had collected broke into a spontaneous cheer, and Coué – slipping modestly away – returned to the fresh company of sufferers who awaited him within.

*SIMPLE SELF-HEALING*

# UNDERSTANDING THE AUTOSUGGESTION METHOD

*TAUGHT BY ÉMILE COUÉ*

*"Conscious autosuggestion – made with confidence, faith and perseverance – realizes itself automatically, in all matters within reason."*

## THE REALITY OF AUTOSUGGESTION

I wish to say how glad I was to come into personal contact with the great American public on their own side of the Atlantic. And, at the same time, I couldn't help feeling just a little embarrassed. I get the idea that people on that continent expected from me some wonderful revelation, bordering on the miraculous…whereas, in reality, the message I have to give is so simple that many are tempted at first to consider it as almost insignificant.

Let me say right here, however, that simple as my message may be, it will teach those who consent to hear it – and to give it fair thought – a key to physical and moral wellbeing which can't be lost.

To the uninitiated, autosuggestion – or self-mastery – is likely to appear disconcerting in its simplicity. But doesn't every discovery, every invention, seem simple and ordinary if it's been presented superficially, without its true substance? Not that I'm claiming autosuggestion as my discovery. Far from it! Autosuggestion is as old as the hills – only we had forgotten to practice it, and so we needed to learn it all over again.

Think of all the forces of the universe ready to serve us. Yet centuries often elapsed before man penetrated their secret and discovered the means of utilizing them.

It's the same in the domain of thought and mind: We have at our service forces of transcendent value, of which we are either completely ignorant, or else only vaguely conscious.

*"The means employed by 'healers' of all eras has been based upon autosuggestion. That's to say that those methods, whatever they are – words, incantations, gestures, staging – all have been designed to produce in the patient the autosuggestion of recovery."*

## POWER OF AUTOSUGGESTION KNOWN THROUGHOUT HISTORY

The power of thought, of idea, is inconceivable and immeasurable. The world is dominated by thought. The human being individually is also *entirely* governed by his own thoughts, good or bad. The powerful action of the mind over the body – which explains the effects of suggestion – was well known to the great thinkers of the Middle Ages, whose vigorous intelligence embraced the sum of human knowledge.

Every idea conceived by the mind, said Saint Thomas, is an order which the organism obeys. It can also, he added, *engender a disease* or *cure it*.

The effectiveness of autosuggestion couldn't be more plainly stated.

We know, indeed, that the whole human organism is governed by the nervous system, the center of which is the brain, the seat of thought. In other words, the brain – or mind – controls every cell, every organ, and every function of the body. That being so, isn't it clear that *by means of thought* we're the absolute masters of our physical organism? And that, as the Ancients showed centuries ago, thought – or suggestion – can and does produce disease or cure it?

Pythagoras taught the principles of autosuggestion to his disciples. He wrote: "God the Father, deliver them from their sufferings, and show them what supernatural power is at their call."

Even more definite is the doctrine of Aristotle, which taught that "a vivid imagination compels the body to obey it, for it is a natural principle of movement. Imagination, indeed, governs all the forces of sensibility, while the latter, in its turn, controls the beating of the heart, and through it sets in motion all vital functions; thus the entire organism may be rapidly modified. Nevertheless, however vivid the imagination, it cannot change the form of a hand or foot or other member."

I've particular satisfaction in recalling this element of Aristotle's teaching, because it contains two of the most important – or, I should say – *essential* principles of my own method of autosuggestion:

1. *The dominating role of the imagination.*

2. *The results to be expected from the practice of autosuggestion must necessarily be limited to those coming within the bounds of physical possibility.*

I'll deal with these essential points in greater detail in another chapter.

Unfortunately, all these great truths, handed down from antiquity, have been transmitted in the cloudy garb of abstract notions – or shrouded in the mystery of esoteric secrecy – and therefore have appeared inaccessible to the ordinary person. However, if I've had the privilege of discerning the hidden meaning of old philosophers – or extracting the essence of a vital principle – and of formulating it in a manner extremely simple and comprehensible to modern humanity, I've also had the greater joy of *seeing it practiced with success* by thousands of sufferers for more than twenty years.

*"Autosuggestion is an instrument which you have to learn how to use, just like any other instrument. An excellent gun in inexperienced hands gives wretched results."*

## SLAVES OF SUGGESTION
## AND MASTERS OF OURSELVES

Please mark and remember these words: *I am no healer*. I can only teach others to cure themselves and to maintain perfect health.

I hope to show you, moreover, that the domain of application of autosuggestion is practically unlimited. Not only are we able to control and modify our physical functions, but we can develop in any desired direction our moral and mental faculties, merely by the proper exercise of autosuggestion.

From our birth to our death, we're all the slaves of suggestion. Our destinies are decided by suggestion. It's an all-powerful tyrant which, unless we take heed, we're the blind instruments. Now, it's in our power to turn the tables and to discipline suggestion, and direct it in the way we ourselves wish. Then it becomes *autosuggestion*. We can take the reins into our own hands, and become masters of the most marvelous instrument conceivable. Nothing then is impossible to us – except, of course, that which is contrary to the laws of nature and the universe.

How are we to attain this command? We must first grasp at least the elements of the mental portion of the human being. Our mental personality is composed of *the conscious* and *the subconscious*. It's generally believed that the power and acts of a man depend almost exclusively upon his conscious self. It's beginning to be understood, however, that compared with the immensity of the role of the subconscious, the conscious self is like a little islet in a vast ocean – subject to storm and tempest.

*"The subconscious self directs everything, both the physical and the moral."*

## DOMINANCE OF THE
## SUBCONSCIOUS OVER THE CONSCIOUS

Symbolically, the subconscious is a permanent, ultra-sensitive photographic plate which nothing escapes. It registers all things, all thoughts, from the most insignificant to the most sublime. But it's more than that. It's the source of creation and inspiration; it's the mysterious power that germinates ideas and effects their materialization in the conscious form of action.

If we agree that the point of departure for our joys, our sorrows, our ills, our well-being, our aspirations – of all our emotions – is in our subconscious self, then we may logically deduct that every idea germinated in our mind has a tendency for realization.

Hundreds of examples drawn from little incidents of everyday existence enable us to verify the truth of all this. To illustrate action of thought on the emotive faculties, we only have to remember any grave accident or harrowing spectacle of which we've been a witness, to immediately *feel* the sensations of pain or horror – with greater or less intensity, according to our individual temperament.

A simpler and perhaps even more striking example is the classic one of the lemon. Imagine that you're sucking a juicy, sour lemon…and your mouth will inevitably and instantaneously begin to water. What's happened? Simply this: Under the influence of the idea, the glands have gone to work and secreted an abundant quantity of saliva – almost as much, in fact, as if you'd actually taken a bite of a real lemon.

Or just think of a scratching chalk pencil being drawn perpendicularly over a blackboard – and you can't avoid shuddering and screwing up your face under the shock, while contracted nerves send a shiver from the back of the head all down your spine.

We must, therefore, realize *that it's impossible to separate the physical from the mental, the body from the mind* – that they are dependent upon each other, that they're really one.

The mental element, however, is always dominant. Our physical body is governed by it. So we actually make or mar our own health and destinies according to the ideas at work in our subconscious. I mean by this that we're absolutely free to implant *whatever* ideas we desire in our subconscious self – which is a never-flagging recorder – and those ideas determine the whole trend of our material, mental, and moral being.

It's just as easy to whisper into our receptive subconscious self the idea of health, as it is to moan over our troubles. And those who do may be certain of the result, because – as I hope I've shown you – it's based on nature's laws.

*"The key to my method is to know that the imagination is superior to the will."*

## THE ROLE OF THE IMAGINATION

Before explaining the practical application of autosuggestion, and the extremely simple method by which it's possible for everyone to gain mastery over his or her physical organism, I must speak of the all-important role of the imagination. Specifically, of the dominance of the imagination over the will.

Contrary to the generally accepted theory, the will *isn't* the invincible force it's claimed to be. In fact, whenever imagination and will come into conflict it is *always* imagination that triumphs.

Try to do something while repeating: *"I can't do it, I can't do it, I can't do it..."*

You'll quickly see this truth confirmed for yourself. The mere *idea* of inability to accomplish a thing paralyzes the willpower.

Self-mastery, therefore, is attained when the imagination has been directed and trained to conform with our desires. For although, in one sense, the imagination is disposed to the subconscious, it really dominates the latter. And, if we know how to guide it, our subconscious self will take charge of our material being and do its work just as we wish it to be done. Or, in other words: *Exactly in conformity with our conscious suggestions.*

I cannot too strongly insist that, in the practice of

autosuggestion, the exercise of willpower must be *strictly avoided*, except in the initial phase of directing or guiding the imagination on the desired lines. This is absolutely the only manifestation of will necessary, or even desirable. Any other voluntary effort is positively harmful in connection with autosuggestion, and will almost certainly have an effect *contrary* to the one desired.

Analyze the so-called "strong-willed" characters of history: Caesar, Napoleon, etc. You'll find that they were all men of *big imagination*. Certain ideas were implanted in their minds, and their tenacious suggestions impelled them into action (this, however, is a slight digression.)

*"People are always preaching the doctrine of effort, but this idea must be repudiated. Effort means will. And will means the possible entrance of the imagination in opposition of the desire, bringing about exactly the contrary result of the desired outcome."*

## LAW OF CONVERTED EFFORT

What I want to drive home is the law that my friend Charles Baudouin calls *"converted effort."*

Suppose a man suffering from insomnia decides to try the effect of autosuggestion. Unless previously warned, he'll repeat to himself phrases like this: *"I want to sleep, I will sleep, I am going to sleep..."* And all the time he'll be making desperate efforts to coax sleep. That's fatal. The very fact of exerting effort has converted the latter into a force acting in a sense *contrary* to the original suggestion, with the result that the poor man tosses and turns in his bed in wretched sleeplessness.

The imagination should be left unhindered.

Let it do its work alone – unhindered. *Be quite passive.* Through mysterious, still unexplained processes our subconscious self accomplishes marvelous things.

Think of the most common movements of the human body and ask yourself how they're operated. What has set in motion the complicated mechanism when you stretch your arm to reach a glass on a table, or when you take a coin from your pocket? No one knows. But even if we cannot explain the phenomenon, we do know that, in actual fact, it's an order resulting from a mere suggestion – which is transmitted through the nervous system, and translated into action at a speed infinitely greater than that of lightning.

*"Contrary to popular belief, it's not our will that makes us act, but our imagination."*

## EXAMPLES OF THE POWER OF IMAGINATION

Thousands of examples of the power of imagination may be found in everyday life. There is the one given by Pascal, and often cited, which I cannot help repeating here, because it's such a perfect illustration: No one would have the slightest difficulty in walking along a foot-wide plank placed on the ground. But put the same plank across a street at the height of one of your American skyscrapers. Even the old French hero Blondel wouldn't have dared trust himself on it! Anyone who did would assuredly fall to death.

No clearer proof of the power of an idea could be desired.

There is, however, a striking complementary example: The impunity with which sleepwalkers perform the most dangerous feats – such as wandering about on a roof, hugging the extreme edge of it, to the terror of their friends who may happen to see them. If awakened suddenly, a sleepwalker in such a position would inevitably fall.

Here's another: Doctor Pinaud, in his book "De la Philosophie et de la Longévité," relates that in the middle of a large dinner party, the cook rushed in to announce that she had made a mistake and mixed arsenic with the food instead of some other ingredient! Several people were immediately seized with pains and sickness, which only ceased when the cook came back to say that it was a false alarm: There had been no such dreadful error!

I've said enough to prove the *irresistible influence* of the idea – or imagination – over the physical body. It determines pain, movement, emotions, and sensations. Its effect is both moral and physical.

We may then logically conclude that human ailments – which are nothing but disturbances of the natural equilibrium of all the elements of our being – can be cured by the right kind of idea or suggestion.

*"Don't spend your time thinking of illnesses and symptoms you might have – for if you have no real ones, you'll create artificial ones."*

## THE MORAL FACTOR IN ALL DISEASE

There is in every disease – no matter what type – a moral factor which no doctor can afford to ignore. Some in France estimate this moral factor represents *40 to 50 percent* of the chance, or speed, of recovery.

In short, a patient who says to himself *"I am getting better"* vastly increases his vital forces and hastens his recovery. By gently putting our imagination on the right track, we're sure of aiding nature, who manifests herself through the medium of our subconscious self.

The instinct of self-preservation is a natural manifestation of nature. At the first sound of alarm, she hastens to the rescue. A cut finger or other wound is followed by a rush of red globules to the injured part. That wonderful subconscious self of ours does it. For it knows and commands every movement of our being, every contraction of our heart, the minutest vibration of every cell in our body. It's the sublime instrument which we're so apt to misuse by allowing bad, disturbing, or discouraging thoughts to interfere with its work – instead of allowing it to function smoothly and harmoniously.

Miracles are often attributed to the Fakirs of India. Legend or fact, I don't know, but it's certainly true that they do some most wonderful things simply because they're taught from their infancy to know – and make use of – the limitless unseen and yet unexplained forces latent in us, which can be awakened by thought.

*"It is not in me but in yourself that you must have confidence. For it's in you alone that dwells the force which can cure you. My part simply consists in teaching you to make use of that force."*

I'm often asked: What are the limitations of autosuggestion? I reply:

*I really don't know.*

The cures I've seen have sometimes appeared so amazing, so incredible, that I decline theoretically to place any limit at all. Although, of course, I insist: Nothing must be expected from autosuggestion which is obviously outside the domain of material possibilities. For instance, it would be absurd to ask for the growth of a new arm or a new leg – despite the fact that the lobster seems to know how to grow a new claw when it's necessary!

There are people who, by long practice and concentration, have acquired an amazing power over their bodily functions. Cases are known to the medical faculty in Paris of men able to increase the speed of their heartbeats from 90 to 120, or diminish it to such a degree that the heart seems almost to stop.

In another chapter, I'll talk of the diseases actually cured by autosuggestion, and its general sphere of curative possibilities. But let it be thoroughly realized that thought – or suggestion – is able to mold the human body as a sculptor chisels his clay.

*Thought is an act.*

It's more than Bernheim believed when he wrote, "Suggestion is an idea which can be transformed into action." It's certain that cases declared to be incurable have been cured by autosuggestion, and not only diseases of a functional nature. Sores and wounds of long standing, which had resisted all other treatments, have been healed rapidly by suggestion. (Was it not Doctor Carnot who said "the wounds of victorious soldiers heal more rapidly than those of the vanquished"?)

I can declare without hesitation that whatever the illness, the practice of rational autosuggestion will always effect an appreciable improvement in the patient's condition, even if the disease itself is incurable.

*"Simplify always – do not complicate."*

## AUTOSUGGESTION IN PRACTICE

After the explanations of the theory of autosuggestion, you're certainly anxious to be initiated in the method of putting it into actual practice. We've seen that our physical body is completely dominated by our subconscious self which, obeying every suggestion – of no matter what nature – transmits it as an order to every fiber of the body, and that the latter responds or reacts immediately.

The only obstacle to the perfect accomplishment of the operation is the intervention of the conscious will, or reason, at the same time. What we want to know, therefore, is the mechanisms by which we may acquire control of our subconscious self – in other words, achieve self-mastery.

The method is simplicity itself. So simple that it's been scoffed at, as all simple solutions of seemingly complicated problems have been scoffed at. But its logic is irrefutable, and its effects are demonstrated every day of our lives.

*All that's necessary is to place oneself in a condition of mental passiveness, silence the voice of conscious analysis, and then deposit in the ever-awake subconscious the idea – or suggestion – which one desires to be realized.*

Every night, when you've comfortably settled yourself

in bed, and are at the point of dropping off to sleep, murmur in a low but clear voice, just loud enough to be heard by yourself, this little formula: *"Every day, in every way, I am getting better and better."*

Recite the phrase like a litany, twenty times or more. And in order to avoid distracting your attention by the effort of counting, it's an excellent idea to tick the number off on a piece of string tied in twenty knots.

"Ridiculous!" you say. Perhaps, yet it suffices to set in motion in the desired direction the stupendous forces of which we may be masters if we do. It's a mere suggestion, but that suggestion cast into the mysterious laboratory of the subconscious self is instantaneously translated into an active, living force.

The Ancients well knew the power – often the terrible power – contained in the repetition of a phrase or a formula. The secret of the undeniable influence they exercised through the old Oracles resided probably – or I should say – *certainly* in the force of suggestion. Yes, my method of self-cure – by autosuggestion – is undoubtedly simple. It's easy to understand and just as easy to practice. Yet the human mind is today what it was in the days of the Oracles: It insists on associating the healing of the body or mind with complicated theories and processes – which, in reality, is quite unnecessary.

*Why complain if things are made easy for you?*

People may wonder why I'm content to prescribe such a general – and apparently vague – formula as *"Every day, in every way, I'm getting better and better"* for all and every ailment. The reason is, strange as it may seem, that our subconscious mind *doesn't* need the details. The general suggestion that everything "in every way" is going well is quite sufficient to set up the procedure of persuasion, which will carry its effects to the different organs and improve every function.

I've had remarkable demonstration of this in the course of my long teaching and experiments. Time and time again, I've seen patients cured not only of the particular disease for which they sought relief, but also of minor disabilities which they had almost forgotten.

*"It isn't the person who acts, it's the method."*

## DON'T CONCENTRATE

The fact is, our subconscious knows *much more* than we can ever know ourselves about our physical organism.

Fortunately for us!

Just think what a mess we should make of things if we had to look after every function – breathing and digestion, for instance. Who is it that takes charge of such a complicated job? The subconscious mind. And if it ever does its work badly, it's always because – in some way or another – we've voluntarily meddled with it.

Every organ or function is connected with – and depends to some degree – upon others. And if the ordinary man or woman were to begin ordering the subconscious tinkering with a particular organ, he or she would certainly be obeyed…only the chances are that something else would then go wrong as a result of insufficient knowledge, or perhaps complete ignorance of physiology on the part of the conscious mind.

So just leave it to the subconscious!

*Avoid all effort.*

When you recite your phrase, *"Every day, in every way, I am getting better and better,"* you must relax all strain and tension. Don't seek to concentrate your thoughts. Concentration is very valuable and necessary when conscious reasoning is to be done, but fatal to the success of autosuggestion.

However, please do isolate yourself from everything likely to distract your attention. Close your eyes if possible. You can obtain mental isolation in a crowd or in a streetcar if need be, and there's no reason why you shouldn't practice autosuggestion in such conditions during the daytime – provided you succeed in putting yourself in the right state of passiveness.

At the risk of being accused of tedious repetition, I must insist on the necessity of passiveness and inertia. Don't think you need to struggle to impose your suggestion. The very fact of making it an effort will bring into play the conscious will, and that willpower actually raises a barrier between the subconscious and the suggestion – and *prevents* the latter from penetrating.

Now, because of what I've said on the superiority of a general formula of autosuggestion, it must not be thought that I altogether discourage the application of suggestion to specific complaints. On the contrary: It's to be *recommended unreservedly* in all cases where it's desired to relieve pain, correct functional disorders, or alleviate their symptoms.

*"We repeat, rapidly and often, that the thing is going to happen, or isn't going to happen, according as to whether it's something desirable or undesirable."*

## HOW TO BANISH PAIN

For such purposes, here's my procedure: To cause pain to vanish, rub the affected spot lightly but rapidly with your hand, at the same time repeating in an undertone – so swiftly as to make it a mere gabble – the words *"Ça passe"* (pronounce "sah pass.") In a few minutes the pain should disappear, or at the very least, be considerably diminished.

The reason for *gabbling* the words is to avoid the risk of any other extraneous or contrary thought slipping in through fissures, which might result from a more distinct but slower diction. It's fine for English-speaking people to stick to the French version, or to say the translation they find most comfortable saying quickly: *"it passes," "it's passing," "it goes,"* or *"it's going."*

*"The repetition of the same words forces us to think them, and when we think them they become true for us, and transform themselves into reality."*

## HOW TO GO TO SLEEP

Sufferers from sleeplessness will proceed in another way: Having settled themselves comfortably in bed they will repeat (not gabble), *"I am going to sleep, I am going to sleep, I am going to sleep..."* in a quiet, placid, even voice – avoiding, of course, the slightest mental effort to attain the desired result.

The soporific effect of this droning repetition of the suggestion soon makes itself felt. Whereas, if one actually *tries* to sleep, the spirit of wakefulness is kept alive by the negative idea, according to the law of converted effort. Insomnia indeed affords a striking demonstration of the disastrous effect of the exertion of the will, the result of which is just the contrary to the one desired.

*"The fear of failure is almost certain to cause failure, just as the very idea of success brings success and enables one to overcome any obstacle in the way."*

## STAMMERING, LACK OF CONFIDENCE AND PARALYSIS CURED

Stammering, again, is a painful affliction which read-ily yields to autosuggestion. I've known cases of cures being affected in one sitting – though this, naturally, is rare. What is the cause of stammering? Merely *the fear* or *the idea* that one is going to stammer. If you can sub-stitute for that idea the conviction, or the suggestion, that you're not going to stutter – that if you can say ten words without stuttering, there's no reason why you should stumble over the eleventh – then you're cured.

Nervousness, timidity, lack of confidence, and even worse nervous phenomena can be eradicated by the practice of autosuggestion. For they're simply the consequences of self-suggestion of a wrong, unnatural character. Those who suffer from such infirmities must set up a different train of suggestions by saying things like, *"I'm not nervous, I'm well and full of confidence, all is going well..."* Likewise, in a fit of anger, try the effect of suddenly murmuring *"I'm calm,"* and you'll be surprised.

There are quite a number of cases of paralysis which are due only to the patient's belief in his or her inability to use the affected limb or member. They can all be cured

– easily, certainly. Implant the notion: *"I can walk, I can move my arm (or leg, or finger),"* and the cure is accomplished.

Why is this? Because although the lesion which originally produced the paralysis has healed already, the patient has lost the habit of using his limb, and still *thinks* he's unable to do so. It's obvious that as strong as that subconscious notion may be, that of a contrary notion must be at least equally strong to be effective. If the *proper* suggestion can be conveyed to the subconscious mind instead of the *improper* suggestion…that's the whole secret.

*"Many, who have had medical treatments their whole life, expect to be cured at once by autosuggestion. That's a mistake. It's unreasonable to expect anything like that. It's useless to ask more of autosuggestion than what it can usually bring about, which is to say: A progressive improvement which slowly transforms itself into a complete recovery, if the latter is at all natural."*

## DISEASES THAT CAN BE CURED

L et's now talk a little about specific diseases which can be cured by autosuggestion. I must repeat what I've said previously: That it's very difficult to place any limit to the powers of autosuggestion (within the bounds of possibility, of course.) For, even in cases of maladies described as incurable, I've had occasion to observe such extraordinary improvement in the patient's condition that the most extravagant hopes *would* seem justified.

It can be affirmed without hesitation that even organic disorders come within the influence of autosuggestion. I'm aware that this contradicts the theory of a number of doctors who, perhaps, judge the matter rather too hastily. But my affirmation is supported by many other eminent members of the fraternity in France and elsewhere who have found its truth demonstrated by actual facts.

Doctor Vachet, professor at the School of Psycho-Therapeutics at Paris, and a distinguished member of the growing corps of physicians who have begun to employ autosuggestion and suggestion as an adjunct to the ordinary resources of medicine, cited recently the case of a young woman cured of ulcers in the stomach by the new method. There was no diagnostic error. X-ray photographs had been taken. A surgical operation had been prescribed. By means of suggestion, unaided by drugs or other treatment, the patient was cured within two months. In the first week, the vomiting had ceased.

The same practitioner mentions the rapid disappearance of a tumor on the tenth rib, the sufferer being a young girl who was also afflicted with a fissure of the anus. The girl had been ill for two years, and in bed for three months. Her temperature was high, and her general condition bad. The power of suggestion cured her in a fortnight, the tumor disappearing completely and the fissure healing without leaving a trace.

Let me show you an example of how symptoms may be cured even when the disease itself may not. In the course of my own experience, one of the most remarkable cases which I can call to mind is that of a boy who, if not actually cured of a serious heart affection – endocarditis – at least got rid of all the symptoms, and lives and enjoys life as though in perfect health.

One day the door of my study was opened and a pale, thin youth entered, leaning heavily on the arm of his father. At every step he paused, and every breath he took was like the painful gasp of an exhausted animal. Poor little chap! I didn't expect to be able to do much for him. However, after his father had explained his malady I took him in hand, demonstrating the force of autosuggestion by means of a few simple experiments such as I usually make during my lectures. For instance, I made him clasp his hands tightly, and then showed him that he couldn't unclasp them while thinking and saying, *"I cannot, I cannot…"*

The boy was convinced. He went away full of confidence, promising to recite my formula regularly and to practice conscientiously the principles of autosuggestion. I saw him a few weeks afterward. There was already a considerable change. He could walk better and his breathing was easier, but he was still in a pitiful condition.

The lad persevered, however, and he did, indeed, "get better and better every day" – and when I heard of him next he was playing football! He was exempted from military service during the war, for medical examination showed him to be still suffering from his heart trouble – although to all intents and purposes he was a well-grown, muscular young man. Which proves that symptoms can always be relieved by autosuggestion, even when the disease itself is incurable.

Take diabetes. According to certain modern authorities, this affection may sometimes have its origin in nervous trouble. Generally, of course, it's organic. In any case, I've known it frequently to yield to autosuggestion practiced with perseverance. Recently, a patient succeeded in reducing the amount of sugar from 80 grams to 59 in less than a month, while several painful symptoms disappeared.

Similarly, without venturing to declare that tuberculosis can be cured by autosuggestion, I do say that in many cases it can be fought successfully. By the practice of autosuggestion, the resistance of the organism is strengthened, and the patient aids nature's own tendency to react against disease.

*This is true, indeed, in all cases of general debility.*

I know a lady of sixty who had been ailing for the better part of her life, and who, when she came to me first, believed she was near death. She weighed barely ninety-eight pounds. Autosuggestion transformed her. The idea of health implanted in her subconscious gave her self-confidence unknown to her previously. Her health improved to such an extent that she recovered from an attack of pulmonary congestion, which her doctor believed she couldn't possibly resist, and she has increased her weight by twenty-six pounds.

Sciatica, gastric troubles, constipation, asthma, and headaches readily give way to autosuggestion. There's a man who had suffered from headaches for thirty years, taking aspirin and similar drugs regularly on certain days of the week. (Notice the power of suggestion: He was convinced he would have a headache on such and such a day, and he did have one.) Now he's set his mind working along other lines, and has cured himself of his chronic headaches.

I also know a man who suffered from sciatica, and who, according to a letter which he wrote the other day, has had practically no pain since the day he came to hear me explain the practice of autosuggestion. And a young woman who now thinks nothing of walking eight miles, although by her doctor's orders she had considered herself an "invalid" for many years, scarcely daring to stir from her bed or her sofa.

Astonishing as these results may appear, they're perfectly logical and natural – since it's been demonstrated that, in certain conditions, wasted tissue may be repaired by the exercise of autosuggestion.

And now, here's a word of comfort to those who are fearful (and how many aren't?) of losing their good looks. Of course, you're right to want to remain young and fresh and good-looking. And you can do so if you only realize that *you* possess the secret yourselves. It's that little fairy who dwells in your subconscious and who asks nothing better than to smooth away those impertinent wrinkles, to put firm cushions of healthy flesh under sagging cheeks, or restore the laughing sparkle to dulled eyes.

Yes, just train your imagination to visualize your face or body as you would like it to be, and you'll have a very good chance of seeing them approach pretty near your ideal. Mind, I don't tell you that you can change the color of your eyes or hair, or modify the shape of your chin or nose – we must always keep to the materially possible. But you can really improve your appearance, and ward off the attacks of age and fatigue.

Fatigue, by the way, ought not to be possible if you practice autosuggestion. It's so largely a matter of imagination. Suppose you have a task to perform. If you think to yourself beforehand, *"this is going to be difficult and tiring,"* it surely will be so, and you'll yawn over it and feel quite tired and bored.

But if you're in a different frame of mind, and say, *"This is going to be easy, I shall enjoy doing it,"* then you'll not feel the slightest trace of fatigue. The best way of making a hard job easy is to buckle down and do it.

*"Contrary to popular opinion, physical diseases are generally more easily cured by autosuggestion than mental ones."*

## ONE MUST OBSERVE THE
## ORDINARY RULES OF HEALTH

It goes without saying that the practice of autosuggestion will not dispense one from the observance of the ordinary rules of health and hygiene. Remember, we're using the forces of nature, so it would be silly to attempt to fight them at the same time.

Lead a rational life. Don't overeat. Chew your food thoroughly. Take sufficient exercise. Avoid excesses. They are nature's laws. Their observance, combined with the knowledge of the all-powerful effects of autosuggestion, will keep you in good physical and moral health, and enable you to combat successfully any of the ills to which the human body is heir through tradition and heredity.

Let me add most emphatically that I don't advise you to dispense with a doctor's services. Obviously, there are many cases in which his advice and medicine and care are absolutely indispensable.

And always, a doctor's presence and prestige and cheering words are helpful to the patient – especially if he also takes advantage of the wonderful instrument at his disposition, and accompanies his prescription with the proper suggestions. The results will be attained with much greater rapidity. I want both patients and doctors to understand that autosuggestion is a most formidable weapon against disease.

*"It's an illusion to think you have no illusions."*

## MORAL POWER OF AUTOSUGGESTION

Leaving for a while the subject of the physical cures affected by autosuggestion, let's discuss the role in relation to our moral well-being. "Train up a child in the way he should go, and when he is old he will not depart from it," said the Man of Wisdom thousands of years ago; and his words are as true now as they were then.

And what is such "training" if not the art of implanting a mass of suggestions in the young, receptive mind? Those suggestions may be good or bad, and upon them depends the child's whole destiny.

I'd like to insist upon the importance of suggestion and autosuggestion for society. Moral health is essential to physical health, and it's to the interest of the community at large to improve the moral health of its feebler elements. Given the efficacy of autosuggestion in the accomplishment of this task, it must be clear that the method opens up a magnificent vista of possibilities in the direction of social progress.

Autosuggestion furnishes us the means of combating victoriously the bad streaks in our nature – whether inherited or acquired – and of developing our intelligence, of curbing a wayward imagination, of adding balance to our judgment, modifying our mentality, correcting our moral weaknesses…all while curing our bodily ills.

*"To be master of yourself, it's enough to think you are the master. And in order to think it, you must repeat it often, without any effort."*

## PSYCHIC CULTURE AS NECESSARY AS PHYSICAL

We all recognize the value of physical culture. It's not too much to say that its revival in my own country – and the consequent building up of a generation of robust, strong limbed young men, full of stamina and resistance – contributed a considerable measure to our victory in the Great War.

Well, psychic culture is equally necessary. It will teach us to think simply, sanely. It'll teach us to realize that we can be, and should be, the masters of events, and not their playthings.

*Psychic culture, through the medium of suggestion and autosuggestion, corrects our moral deformities, just as physical culture corrects our bodily defects.*

To people who ask if vice really can be conquered, I answer emphatically yes. By suggestion – *long and oft repeated* – the character can be modified. Suggestion too often acts as a break to bad instincts – that's its negative role. It has a positive part to play in acting as a propelling force for good impulses. Applied systematically, particularly through positive autosuggestion, there's no doubt that a large portion of the classes branded as "criminal" could be reclaimed, and thousands of outcasts transformed into clean-thinking, clean living, and useful citizens.

This is, naturally, especially true regarding the young – with their keen, vigorous imaginations open to every impression. Surely it's the duty of those in authority to see that their imagination be fed with something better than the germs of crime. The susceptibility of youth is such that it's easy (save in the rare cases of wholly bad characters) to create vivid images or ideas of good actions in their minds. Once anchored in the subconscious, those ideas must inevitably develop and eventually externalize themselves in acts.

*"Let us be calm, gentle, benevolent, sure of ourselves – and moreover, let us be self-sufficient."*

## EDUCATION OF CHILDREN

Paradoxical as it may appear to those who haven't fully understood the principles and workings of autosuggestion, the education of a child begins even before it's born!

Without going back to explanations which I have given, I need only say that the imagination plays the supreme role in every function of life, and that by disciplining it – in other words, by exercising autosuggestion – a prospective mother can not only determine the sex of her child (this has been demonstrated by certain medical authorities) but also, to a large degree, its physical and moral characteristics. She has only to let her imagination deposit in her subconscious mind the image of the son or daughter she desires and the qualities she wishes the unborn infant to possess. The result is assured.

Even more important, perhaps, is the fact that such a child will yield more readily than most to suggestion. Which doesn't mean that its character is likely to be weak. On the contrary, the probabilities are that it will – as it grows up – exchange suggestion for autosuggestion, and achieve perfect self-mastery. Only it must be remembered that our acts and deeds are, for the most part, the result of past outside suggestions or example.

The importance of beginning a child's education early,

and of controlling the suggestions destined to influence and mold the young mind, must therefore be obvious. Parents and educators must be careful to implant in it only good suggestions and protect it at all costs from bad ones.

How's that done? I'll try to give a few recommendations. They must, of course, be taken as general ones, and may be modified or adapted to individual subjects and circumstances. Treat children with an equitable temper, speaking in tones gentle but firm, persuading them to obey without giving them the temptation to resist your influence. Never be rough with a child, for to do so is to risk provoking a sentiment of fear accompanied by sullenness or even hate. Avoid talking ill of people in the presence of children; they'll inevitably follow your example later on. And backbiting often leads to disaster.

Seek to awaken in children's minds the desire to understand nature. Keep them interested. Answer their questions clearly, with good-humor. Don't put them off – as so many of us are tempted to do – with such replies as, "Oh, you're bothering me," or "You'll know all about that later." Above all, never on any account tell a child that he or she is a "storyteller," or lazy, or a dunce, or worse. Remember that such suggestions have a very strong tendency to become realities, just as the better kinds of suggestions have.

Encouragement is particularly necessary to children. Say to a child inclined to be lazy or negligent, "Well, you've done much better than usual today. I'm very pleased with your work, you're improving." It may not be true. No matter. The idea of improvement – of excellence, of endeavor – will sink into the child's mind and gradually, with judicious encouragement, be transformed unconsciously into fact.

Avoid discussing diseases before children – autosuggestion is quick to carry the idea to the physical plane and develop the very illness you wish to avert. Teach them, on the contrary, that good health is normal – and sickness is an anomaly and aberration which is only a consequence of the non-observance of nature's laws.

Never frighten children. Don't let a child fear the elements. Man is made to stand cold, heat, rain, etcetera without ill effects; it's merely an idea that creates weakness. Likewise, it's a cruel thing to frighten children by talking of "bogies" and goblins and the like; fear thus instilled may persist and ruin a child's later life and destiny.

Set only good examples. It's unnecessary, and not in the scope of this chapter, to enumerate all the qualities which a child should possess. All I wish to explain is the employment of suggestion and autosuggestion in a child's education. We all know that "example is better than precept," but we realize the truth of it with greater force after studying the power of autosuggestion. And children are particularly sensitive to suggestion; they're always ready to copy what they see, good or bad. So the first duty of parents and educators is to set only good examples.

Also, suggestion while children are falling asleep may be practiced with wonderful effect, to correct any defect in a child's character, and to develop missing qualities. Every night, just as the child is about to fall off to sleep – or when they're already asleep – stand about a yard away from them, and murmur in a low undertone what you wish to obtain, repeating fifteen to twenty times the qualities desired or the defects to be corrected.

Don't be afraid to repeat the same phrases monotonously. That's the most powerful means of reaching the subconscious. The latter needs no eloquence to be impressed. A plain statement of the idea is sufficient. More than that defeats the ends to be attained.

Character is formed by imagination. In a word, it's essential that a child should be impregnated with the right kind of suggestions. Everything depends upon it. Play upon the imagination – *character is formed by imagination*. More often than not, that which is attributed to heredity – in the moral domain as well as in the physical – is the consequence of ideas germinated by example. It's impossible to believe a child is born a criminal. He becomes one by autosuggestion, just as he may become a valued member of the community as the result of autosuggestion guided in the right direction.

*"Be absolutely certain in your mind that you'll get what you want."*

## MASTERS OF OUR DESTINIES

Monsieur Jourdain, the "Bourgeois Gentilhomme" in Molière's play, "spoke prose without knowing it." In the same way, we all practice autosuggestion, but often without being conscious of it.

To a certain extent, autosuggestion may be automatic, in the sense that it may not be inspired or guided by deliberate reflection. But how much more potent a factor it must be in our lives when we have learned its mechanism, and discovered how to make use of it for our own ends! The act of breathing is automatic – yet we can modify our *manner* of breathing. We can improve our health by learning to breathe in a certain way, and by doing regular breathing exercises. So it is with autosuggestion. Once we realize its force, and learn to control it, we become masters of our destinies.

Babies automatically practice autosuggestion. Let me give you an illustration of this automatic practice. A newborn baby, in its cradle, begins to cry. Immediately, its mother takes it in her arms. The infant stops crying, and then is placed back in the cradle. Whereupon the crying begins all over again, only to stop once more if the baby is lifted from its cradle.

The operation may be repeated an almost unlimited number of times, always with the same result. The child, lacking conscious thought, is automatically practicing autosuggestion. It obtains the gratification of its unconscious desire to be taken into its mother's arms by crying. If resisted, on the other hand – if left to cry alone in its cradle – its subconscious mind will register the fact, and the baby will not take the trouble to cry, because it knows it will have no effect.

Understand that self-mastery means health. And it's like that with everyone, from birth to death. We live by autosuggestion; we're governed by our subconscious mind. Happily, we're able to guide it by our reason. Like everything else, however, the science of autosuggestion has to be learned. It's a matter of educating oneself so that control of the subconscious mind is attained – meaning self-mastery and health.

*"To be afraid of becoming ill is to invite illness."*

## PREVENTION IS BETTER THAN CURE

The idea of good health begets good health, and if by accident we're attacked by disease, we're certain to have an infinitely greater chance of resisting – and of rapidly throwing off the malady – by practicing autosuggestion than if we know nothing of its principles.

Haven't you noticed this during epidemics? It's a well-known fact that people who in such times go serenely about their business – not worrying for themselves, and not giving thought to the epidemic, except to tell themselves that they're sure not to catch the sickness – are almost always immune and escape contagion. On the other hand, nervous people, frightened by the cases around them – and allowing their thoughts to run constantly on the prevailing malady – are certain to fall ill, despite all their precautions.

*"Things which seem miraculous to you have a perfectly natural cause. If they seem extraordinary to you, it's only because the cause escapes you."*

## MODERN MIRACLES

Amazing instances of the power of suggestion are recorded in the annals of the Faculty of Paris. Professor Bouchet relates the following, among many others: An old lady, after undergoing a desperate surgical operation, was dying. Her son was due to arrive from India two days later. Humanly speaking, it was impossible for her to live so long. The method of suggestion was resorted to. She was told that she was better and that she would see her son on the morrow. The result was a complete success. A fortnight later, the old lady was still alive. And, from a medical point of view, that was a miracle.

Equally miraculous, to all appearances, was the case of a man occupying an important position at Nancy a few years ago. He came to me suffering from sinusitis. He had undergone eleven operations, but the terrible disease continued its ravages. He was in a horrible condition, physically and morally. Day and night, without intermission, the unfortunate man was tortured by excruciating pains in the head which prevented him from sleeping. His weakness was extreme, and his appetite nonexistent. Most of the time, he remained helpless on a sofa.

I confess that I had little hope of being able to do

anything for him. However, I took pains to convince him of the efficacy of suggestion. And though there seemed to be no amelioration during five or six sittings, I could see that the man – sick as he was – had gained absolute faith in the soundness of the theories I'd expounded to him. He told me he was daily directing his subconscious mind to the idea of healing his sickness. Then, one day he said he believed that he felt a slight improvement, but wasn't quite sure. It was the truth, however, and the improvement continued. A complete cure followed rapidly. Today that man is perfectly healthy, able to work without fatigue. The discharges from the nose which occurred daily have ceased.

I remember another remarkable case of collective autosuggestion, more or less "automatic" this time. It happened in the hospital services of Doctor Renaud, in Paris. A new serum, an alleged cure for tuberculosis, had just been discovered. It was tested on the patients. Apparently, as a result of the injections, all showed an immediate improvement. The coughing diminished and other symptoms disappeared, and the general condition of all began to be very satisfactory. Alas! Shortly afterward, it became known that the famous serum from which the patients unconsciously hoped for so much was nothing but an ordinary drug, which had been previously tested with negative results. At once, with the fading away of their illusions, the sick men and women lost all the improvement gained, and their old symptoms reappeared.

Miracles happen in our time as they have done in the

past. I mean the things that are called "miracles." For, of course, there's no such thing as a miracle. The modem miracle is worked by autosuggestion – the wonderful force entrusted to us by nature – and which, if we will only probe its mysteries, shall make us all-powerful within the limits of human possibilities. Fatality and fatalism shall lose their meaning. No, they cannot exist, save in our erring imagination. For it's we ourselves who alone shall shape our destinies, rising always above the external circumstances and conditions, which from time to time may be thrown across our paths.

*"We can make, to ourselves, very much stronger suggestions than anyone else can – no matter who that other person may be."*

## I AM NOT A HEALER

When, under the shadow of the Statue of Liberty, I found myself bombarded with questions by a score of newspaper people – who'd come aboard the Majestic specially to meet my humble person – I began to have a faint idea of the interest awakened in America by the announcement of my lecture tour. When I was escorted soon afterward by stalwart American policemen from the ship to the automobile, waiting to convey me to my temporary home with friends – and when I caught sight of the crowds gathered to welcome me – I was inexpressibly surprised and touched that I should be considered worthy of such a reception.

I'm still somewhat dominated by that feeling of surprise which seized me at my first contact with the American people. In fact, my wonderment has grown every day with the realization of the ideas many people seem to have formed of me and my powers.

I don't want people to have a sort of fanatical belief in me. It's true, of course, that blind faith is always an asset in favor of a sick person's chances of getting well. People who come to me with the belief already established in their minds that they're going to be cured are more than halfway on the road to recovery before they see me.

But the number of people who can come into direct contact with me must, of necessity, be relatively small. Even if I possessed any extraordinary magnetic power to heal – *which I emphatically declare I do not* – the results of such power would be limited for obvious reasons. Whereas there are no limitations to the potentialities of the system I teach.

I mean that I cannot personally reach everyone, but everyone can practice autosuggestion. My aim, therefore, is solely to show you how to cure yourselves. Rid yourselves of the utterly wrong idea that I can cure: *I am not a healer.*

*"If there's doubt, there's not results."*

## No Healer or Doctor

I first had an inkling of the mistake America was making when newspaper reporters addressed me as "Doctor" and "Professor" – and I was obliged to correct them with reminders that "I'm not a doctor or a professor." The papers continue to talk of the cures I have effected in my "clinics" – another bad word, by the way, for the little gatherings at which I meet a selected number of patients is in order to convince them *that they can cure themselves*, or at least gain appreciable improvement.

Yes, it's been my joy to see many of these poor sufferers benefit from my teaching. But my joy will be still greater if I succeed in spreading faith in those methods to hundreds of thousands of others, and instill in them the knowledge that they can cure themselves without seeing me at all. And it will be impossible to attain that goal if the impression be allowed to persist that it's necessary to come into personal contact with me in order to obtain results.

Unfortunately, it's very difficult to convince some people that I don't exercise a certain influence over them. When I tell them that they must count upon themselves, not upon me, they often reply: "I don't care what you say, you do wield power, and when I'm with you I get better results than when I'm alone." Well, that may be true in many cases. But the reason, as I've already indicated, is a person who has faith enough to come to me is already half cured by that very faith.

There's another aspect of the question. If I possessed any real power, surely it should have the same effect upon all. Yet that's not the case. Upon some, my influence is absolutely nil. Upon others it may be immense. Which proves that it's not and cannot be an essential factor in the efficacy of my system. My "power" exists merely in the imagination of certain people, as I've explained. The imagination is all powerful, so in such instances it really does aid the recovery of health.

But it would be a sorry action to allow it to be thought that personal contact with me is necessary. I want everyone to understand that all they need is a proper comprehension of the principles of autosuggestion – which is simplicity itself – together with a belief in its effectiveness.

*"Rich is he who thinks he is rich, and poor is he who thinks he is poor."*

AUTOSUGGESTION HAS NO RELATION TO RELIGION

I'm merely applying truths known for thousands of years. I don't claim to have invented anything. I've merely reduced, to a simple formula for everyday use, theories which were known to be truths thousands of years ago.

Still less have I invented a new faith, as some would appear to infer. One day a gentleman, interviewed by one of the newspapers, described my method of autosuggestion as a "direct challenge to the Church."

I confess, I fail to see any relation between religion and autosuggestion.

Is medicine a challenge to the Church? Autosuggestion is only the use of natural forces and functions of our being, and can be practiced by Catholics and Protestants, Muslims or Buddhists, without violating any of the precepts or doctrinal principles of those churches or religions. Didn't Saint Paul write of the "Faith that moved mountains"? Surely it cannot be wrong to make use of the faculties which the Creator himself has given us!

Autosuggestion has no connection with religion. Some religious leaders look suspiciously at autosuggestion because it's come to be associated with alleged "miracles" which I'm supposed to have worked. Now, as I've said, miracles do not exist. I've never accomplished any, and

86

never shall. As a matter of fact, the so-called "miraculous" cures are the simplest and the most easily explained of all. They prove that, actually, the sufferers only *thought* they were sick. Thought produced (or prolonged) the symptoms – and in that respect they were really sick. But directly they were made to realize that their ills could be overcome by imagination, so they were cured.

It may seem rather unnecessary for me to answer the few criticisms of which I've been subject to, in light of the exceptionally sympathetic interest in which I found myself in America. But I'm anxious to clear away all misunderstandings. I wish to be taken seriously by serious-minded people. I want everyone to be convinced that the theories I advance, reduced as they are to their simplest expression, are nevertheless built upon the groundwork of scientific fact.

# ADDITIONAL PRACTICAL NOTES ON AUTOSUGGESTION

## BY CYRUS HARRY BROOKS

*"Always think that what you have to do is easy, if possible."*

## THOUGHT AND WILLPOWER

If we can get the subconscious to accept an idea, realization follows automatically. The only difficulty which confronts us in the practice of induced autosuggestion is to assure acceptation – and that's a difficulty which Émile Coué's method has satisfactorily surmounted.

If upon getting into bed at night, we assume a comfortable posture – relax our muscles and close our eyes – we naturally fall into a state of semi-consciousness akin to that of daydreaming. If we then introduce into the mind a desired idea, it's freed from the inhibiting associations of daily life. It associates itself by similarity, and attracts emotions of the same quality as its own charge. The subconscious is thus caused to accept it, and inevitably it's turned into an effective autosuggestion. Every time we repeat this process, the associative power of the idea is increased, its emotional value grows greater, and the autosuggestion resulting from it is more powerful.

This means we can induce the subconscious to accept an idea – an idea which it normally wouldn't easily accept. The person with a disease-soaked mind can gradually implant ideas of health, filling their subconscious daily with healing thoughts. The instrument we use is thought, and the condition essential to success *is that the conscious mind shall be lulled to rest.*

Systems which up to now have tried to make use of

self-induced suggestion have largely failed to secure reliable results because they didn't place their reliance on thought, but tried to compel the subconscious to accept an idea by exercising willpower. Obviously, such attempts are doomed to failure. By making efforts of willpower we automatically wake ourselves up, suppress the soothing tide of the subconscious, and thereby destroy the condition by which we can succeed.

It's worthwhile to note more closely how this happens. A sufferer, whose mind is filled with thoughts of ill-health, sits down to compel himself to accept a good suggestion. He calls up a thought of health, and makes an effort of the will to impress it on the subconscious. This effort restores him to full wakefulness, and so evokes the customary association—disease. Consequently, he finds himself contemplating the exact *opposite* of what he desired.

He summons his willpower again and recalls the healthful thought, but since he's now wider awake than ever, negative association is even more rapid and powerful than before. The thought of disease is now in full possession of his mind, and all the efforts of his willpower fail to dislodge it. Indeed, the harder he struggles, the more fully the evil thought possesses him.

This gives us a glimpse of the discovery to which Coué's success is due: *That when the will is in conflict with an idea, the idea invariably gains the day.*

This is true, of course, not only of induced autosuggestion, but also of the spontaneous suggestions which occur in daily life. A few examples will make this clear. Most of us know how, when we have some difficult duty to perform, a chance word of discouragement will dwell in the mind, eating away our self-confidence and attuning our minds to failure. All the efforts of our willpower still fail to throw it off – indeed, the more we struggle against it the more we become obsessed by it. Very similar to this is the state of mind of the person suffering from stage-fright. He's obsessed with ideas of failure, and all the efforts of his will are powerless to overcome them. Indeed, it's the state of *effort and tension* which makes his discomfort so complete.

Sports also offer many examples of the working of this law. A tennis player is engaged to play in an important match. He wishes, of course, to win – but fears that he'll lose. Even before the day of the game his fears begin to realize themselves. He is nervy and "out of sorts." In fact, his subconscious is creating the conditions best suited to realize the thoughts in his mind – failure. When the game begins, his skill seems to have deserted him. He summons the resources of his willpower and tries to compel himself to play well, straining every nerve to recapture the old dexterity. But all his efforts only make him play worse and worse. The harder he tries the more he fails. The energy he calls up obeys not his will but the idea in his mind – not the desire to win but the dominant thought of failure.

The fatal attraction of the bunker for the nervous golfer is due to the same cause. With his mind's eye, he sees his golf ball going in the most unfavorable spot. He may use any club he likes, he may make a long drive or a short drive – as long as the thought of the bunker dominates his mind, the ball will inevitably find its way towards it. The more he calls on willpower to help him, the worse his plight is likely to be.

Success is not gained by effort, but by right thinking. The champion golfer or tennis player isn't a person of herculean frame and immense willpower. His whole life has been dominated by *the thought* of success in the game at which he excels.

Students sitting for an examination sometimes undergo this painful experience: On reading through their test, they find that all their knowledge has suddenly deserted them. Their mind is an appalling blank and not one relevant thought can they recall. The more they grit their teeth and summon the powers of the will, the further the desired ideas flee. But later, when they've left the examination room and the tension relaxes, the ideas they were seeking flow tantalizingly back into the mind. Their forgetfulness was due to thoughts of failure previously nourished in the mind. The application of willpower only made the disaster more complete.

This often explains the baffling experience of the drug addict, the alcoholic, or the victim of some other vicious craving. His mind is obsessed by the desire for satisfaction. The efforts of willpower to restrain it only make it *more* overmastering. Repeated failures convince him at length that he's powerless to control himself, and this idea

– operating as an autosuggestion – increases his impotence. So, in despair, he abandons himself to his obsession, and his life ends in wreckage.

We can now see, not only that willpower – in the sense of effort – is incapable of vanquishing a thought, but that as fast as willpower brings up its big guns, thought captures them and turns them against it.

This truth, which Charles Baudouin calls the law of reversed effort (or the law of converted effort), is thus stated by Coué:

*"When the imagination and the will are in conflict, the imagination invariably gains the day."*

Or:

*"In the conflict between the will and the imagination, the force of the imagination is in direct ratio to the square of the will."*

The mathematical terms are used, of course, only metaphorically. Thus, willpower turns out *not* to be the commanding monarch of life – as many people would have it – but a blind Samson, capable either of turning the mill or of pulling down the pillars.

*Autosuggestion succeeds by avoiding conflict.*

It replaces wrong thought by right, literally applying in the sphere of science the principle enunciated in the New Testament: *"Resist not evil, but overcome evil with good."*

This doctrine is in no sense a negation of the will. It simply puts it in its right place, subordinates it to a higher power. A moment's reflection suffices to show that will-power can't be more than the servant of thought. We're incapable of exercising the will unless the imagination has first furnished it with a goal. We cannot simply will – we must will *something*, and that something exists in our minds as an idea.

Willpower acts rightly when it's in harmony with the idea in the mind.

But what happens when, in the smooth execution of our idea, we're confronted with an obstacle? Well, this obstacle may exist outside us – like the golfer's bunker – but it must also exist as an idea *in our minds*, or we wouldn't be aware of it. As long as we allow this negative mental image to stay there, the efforts of our will to overcome it only make it more irresistible. We run our heads against it like a goat butting a brick wall.

Indeed, in this way we can magnify the smallest difficulty until it becomes insurmountable. We can make molehills into mountains. This is precisely what can happen to a deeply anxious or nervous person. The idea of a difficulty dwells unchanged in his mind, and all his efforts to overcome it only increase its dimensions, until it overpowers him – and he faints in the effort to cross a street or do an otherwise simple thing.

But as soon as we *change* the idea, our troubles vanish. By means of the intellect, we can substitute the idea of the obstacle (e.g. "I'm sick") with that of the final solution (e.g. "I'm healthy.") Immediately, willpower is brought into harmony again with thought, and we can go forward towards the triumphant attainment of our end.

It may be that the means adopted to achieve our goal consist of a frontal attack – the overcoming of an obstacle by force. But before we bring this force into play, the mind must have *approved* it – must have positively entertained the idea of its probable success. We must, in fact, have thought of the obstacle as *already* smashed down and flattened out by our attack. Otherwise, we should involve ourselves in the conflict depicted above, and our force would be exhausted in a futile internal battle.

In a forceful attack against an obstacle we use effort, and effort – to be effective – must be *approved* by reason and preceded, to some extent, *by the idea of success.*

Thus, even in our explicit dealings with the outside world, thought is always the master of willpower. And how much more so when our action is turned inward! When practicing autosuggestion, we're living in the mind, where thoughts are the only realities: We can meet with no obstacle other than that of thought itself.

Obviously then, a frontal attack in autosuggestion – the exertion of effort – can never be admissible, for it sets willpower and thought immediately in opposition with each other. In autosuggestion, the turning of our thoughts – from the mere recognition of an obstacle to the idea of the means to overcome it – is no longer necessary, as in the case of outward action. Autosuggestion in itself clears away the obstacle: *By procuring the right idea, our end is already attained.*

So, by applying effort during the practice of induced autosuggestion, we use in the world of mind an instrument fashioned for use in the world of external matter. It's as if we tried to solve a mathematical problem by mauling the book with a tin-opener.

For two reasons, then, effort must never be allowed to intrude during the practice of autosuggestion: First, because it wakes us up and suppresses the gentle tide of the subconscious; secondly, because it causes conflict between thought and willpower.

One other interesting fact emerges from an examination of the previous examples. In each case, we find that the idea which occupied the mind was of a final state – an accomplished fact. The golfer was thinking of his ball dropping unfortunately into the bunker, the tennis player of his defeat, the student of his failure. In each case the subconscious realized the thought in its own way, and chose inevitably the means best suited to arrive at its end – the realization of the negative idea.

In the case of the golfer, the most delicate physical adjustments were necessary. Stance, grip and swing all contributed their part, but these physical adjustments were performed subconsciously – the conscious mind being unaware of them. From this, we see that we don't need to suggest the way in which our aim is to be accomplished. If we fill our mind with *the thought* of the desired end, provided that end is possible, the subconscious will lead us to it by the easiest, most direct path.

Here we catch a glimpse of the truth behind what's

called "luck." We're told that everything comes to him who waits, and this is literally true – provided he waits in the right frame of mind. Some people are notoriously lucky in business; whatever they touch seems to "turn to gold." The secret of their success lies in the fact that they confidently *expect to succeed*.

There's no need to go so far as the school of "New Thought," and claim that suggestion can set in motion transcendental laws outside man's own nature. It's quite clear that the man who expects success – whatever kind it may be – will subconsciously take up the right attitude to achieve it in his environment. He'll involuntarily succeed, even if only fleeting opportunities are presented to him, and by his inner fitness naturally command the circumstances around him.

Man has often been likened to a ship navigating the seas of life. On that ship the engine is the will, and thought is the helm. If we're being directed off our true course, it's worse than useless to call for full steam ahead – our only hope lies in changing the direction of the helm.

*"Don't be afraid to think of your trouble, but say to it, 'I'm not afraid of you.' If you enter a home somewhere and a dog suddenly jumps at you barking, look straight into its eyes and it will not bite you. But if you're afraid and turn your back, it will soon bury its teeth into your leg."*

## SOME GENERAL RULES FOR AUTOSUGGESTION

With our knowledge of the powerful effect which an idea produces, we should see the importance of exercising a more careful censorship over the thoughts which enter our minds.

Thought is the legislative power in our lives, just as willpower is the executive. We don't think it's wise to permit inmates of prisons to occupy legislative posts in the state; yet when we harbor ideas of sin and disease, we allow the criminals and lunatics of thought to usurp the governing power in the commonwealth of our being.

In the future, then, we should seek ideas of health, success, and goodness. We should treat warily all depressing subjects of conversation: The daily list of crimes and disasters which fill the newspapers – as well as those novels, plays and films which disturb our feelings without transmuting, by the magic of their art, sadness into beauty.

This doesn't mean that we should be always self-consciously studying ourselves, ready to nip the pernicious idea in the bud, nor that we should adopt the ostrich's policy of sticking our heads in the sand and declaring that disease and evil have no real existence. One leads to egotism and the other to callousness.

Duty sometimes requires us to give our attention to things in themselves evil and depressing. The demands of friendship and human sympathy are vital, and we cannot ignore them without moral loss.

*But there's a positive and a negative way of approaching such subjects.*

Sympathy is too often regarded as a passive process – by which we allow ourselves to be infected by the gloom, weakness and mental ill-health of other people. This is sympathy perverted. If a friend is suffering from a disease you don't seek to prove your sympathy by infecting yourself with the same disease. You would recognize this to be a crime against the community. Yet many people submit themselves to infection by unhealthy ideas, as if it were an act of charity and part of their duty towards their neighbors.

In the same way, people subject their minds to harrowing stories of war and famine, as if the mental depression thus produced were of some value to the far-away victims. This is obviously false and the only result is to cause gloom and ill-health in the reader, and so make him a burden to his family.

That such disasters should be known is beyond question, but we should react to them in the manner indicated previously. We should replace the passive recognition of the evil by the quest of the means best suited to overcome it. Then we can look forward to an inspiring end, and place the powers of our will in the service of its attainment.

Autosuggestion, far from producing callousness, dictates the method and supplies the means by which the truest sympathy can be practiced. In every case, our aim must be to remove the suffering as soon as possible – and this is facilitated by refusing to accept the bad ideas, and maintaining our own mental and moral balance.

Whenever gloomy thoughts come to us, whether from without or within, we should quietly transfer our attention to something brighter. Even if we're afflicted by some actual malady, we should keep our thought from resting on it as far as we have the power to do so.

An organic disease may be increased a hundredfold by allowing the mind to brood on it, for in so doing we place at its disposal all the resources of our organism, and direct our life-force to our own destruction.

On the other hand, by denying the disease our attention and opposing it with curative autosuggestions, we reduce its power to the minimum and should succeed in overcoming it entirely. Even in the most serious organic diseases, the element contributed by wrong thought is infinitely greater than that which is purely physical.

There are times when temperamental failings – or the gravity of our affliction – places our imagination beyond our ordinary control. Negative suggestions operate in spite of us – we don't seem to possess the power to rid our minds of adverse thoughts. Under these hard conditions, we should *never* struggle to throw out the obsessing idea by force. Our exertions only bring into play the law of reversed effort, and we flounder deeper into the slough. Coué's technique, however, gives us the means of mastering ourselves, even under the most trying conditions.

Of all the destructive suggestions we must learn to shun, none is more dangerous than fear. In fearing something the mind is not only dwelling on a negative idea, but it's establishing the closest personal connection between the idea and ourselves. Moreover, the idea is surrounded by an aura of emotion, which considerably intensifies its effect. Fear combines every element necessary to give a negative autosuggestion its maximum power.

But – happily – fear too is susceptible to the controlling power of autosuggestion. It's one of the first things which a person, cognizant of the means to be applied, should seek to eradicate from their mind through positive autosuggestion.

For our own sake, too, we should avoid dwelling on the faults and frailties of our neighbors. If ideas of selfishness, greed and vanity are continually before our minds, there's great danger that we'll subconsciously accept them, and so realize them in our own character. Petty gossip and backbiting, so common in a small town, produce the very faults they seem to condemn. But by instead allowing our minds to rest upon the virtues of our neighbors, we can reproduce the same virtues in ourselves.

And if we should avoid negative ideas for our own sake, much more should we do so for the sake of other people. Gloomy, despondent men and women are centers of mental contagion, damaging all with whom they come in contact. Sometimes such people involuntarily seem to exert themselves to quench the cheerfulness of brighter natures, as if their subconscious strove to reduce all others to its own low level.

But even healthy, well-intentioned people scatter evil suggestions everywhere, without the least suspicion of the harm they do. Every time we remark to an acquaintance that he's looking ill, we actually damage his health. The effect may be extremely slight, but by repetition it grows powerful.

A person who accepts in the course of a day fifteen or twenty suggestions that he's ill has gone a considerable part of the way towards actual illness. Similarly, when we thoughtlessly commiserate with a friend on the difficulty of their daily work, or represent it as irksome and uncongenial, we make it a little harder for them to accomplish and execute, and thereby slightly diminish their chances of success.

If we must supervise our speech in contact with adults, with children we should exercise still greater foresight. The child's subconscious is far more accessible than that of the adult – the selective power exercised by the conscious mind is much weaker, and consequently the impressions received realize themselves with greater power in a child. These impressions are the material from which the child's growing life is constructed, and if we supply faulty material, the resultant structure will be unstable.

Yet the most attentive and well-meaning mothers are engaged daily in sowing the seeds of weakness in their children's minds! The little ones are constantly told they'll take cold, will be sick, will fall down, or will suffer some other misfortune. The more delicate the child's health, the more likely it's to be subjected to adverse suggestions.

Children are too often saturated with the idea of bad health, and come to look on disease as the normal state of existence, and health as exceptional. The same is equally true of the child's mental and moral upbringing. How often do foolish parents tell their children that they're naughty, disobedient, stupid, lazy or vicious? If these suggestions were accepted – which, thank heaven, isn't always the case – the little ones would very much in fact develop just these qualities.

But even when no word is spoken, a look or a gesture can initiate an undesirable autosuggestion. A child, visited by two strangers, sometimes will immediately make friends with one and avoid the other. Why is this? Because one carries with him a healthful atmosphere, while the other sends out waves of irritability or gloom.

"Men imagine," says Emerson, "that they communicate their virtue or vice only by overt actions, and do not see that virtue and vice emit a breath every moment."

With children, above all, it's not just sufficient to refrain from the expression of negative ideas – we must avoid harboring them altogether. Unless we possess a bright, positive mind the suggestions derived from us will be of little value.

A great deal of what's called hereditary disease is transmitted from parent to child not physically, but mentally – that's to say, by means of adverse suggestions continually renewed in the child's mind. Thus, if one of the parents is constantly sick, the child often lives in an atmosphere laden with thoughts of sickness. The little one is continually advised to take care of their lungs, keep their chest warm, to beware of colds, etc., etc. In other words, the idea is repeatedly presented to its mind that they possess second-rate lungs or other organs. The realization of these ideas, the actual production of a sickly child, is thus almost assured.

But all this is no more than crystallized common sense. Everyone knows that a cheerful mind suffuses health, while a gloomy one produces conditions favorable to disease. "A merry heart doeth good like a medicine," says the writer of the Book of Proverbs, "but a broken spirit drieth the bones."

However, this knowledge – lacking a scientific basis – has never been systematically applied. We've regarded our feelings far too much as *effects* and not sufficiently as *causes*.

We're happy because we're well – we don't recognize that the process works equally in the reverse direction: That we shall be well *because* we're happy.

Happiness is not only the result of our conditions of

life; it is also *the creator* of those conditions. Autosuggestion lays weight upon this latter view. Happiness must come first. It's only when the mind is ordered, balanced – filled with the light of sweet and joyous thought – that it can work with its maximum efficiency. When we're habitually happy, our powers and capabilities come to their full blossom, and we're able to work with the utmost effectiveness on the shaping of what lies around us.

Happiness, they say, can't be ordered like a steak in a restaurant. Like love, its very essence is freedom. This is true. But like love, happiness can be wooed and won. It's a condition which everyone experiences at some time in life. It's native to the mind. By the systematic practice of induced autosuggestion, we can make it not just a fleeting visitant – but a regular tenant of the mind, which external storms and stresses cannot dislodge.

This idea of indwelling happiness, inwardly conditioned, is as ancient as thought. By autosuggestion we can realize it in our own lives.

*"We can lead the imagination along the right path – as indicated by our reason – by consciously employing the mechanical process which we now so often employ unconsciously to lead us the wrong way."*

## <u>ADVANTAGES OF THE GENERAL FORMULA</u>

We saw that a golfer, who imagines his ball going into a bunker, subconsciously performs just those physical movements needed to realize his unfortunate idea in actuality. In realizing this idea, his subconscious displays ingenuity and skill that's admirable – in spite of opposing his stated desire of hitting the ball on the green. From this and other examples we concluded that if the mind dwells on the idea of an accomplished fact, a realized state, the subconscious will produce this state.

If this is true of our spontaneous autosuggestions, it's equally true of the self-induced ones. It follows that if we consistently think of happiness we become happy; if we think of health we become healthy; if we think of goodness we become good. Whatever thought we continually think, provided it's reasonable, tends to become an actual condition of our life.

Traditionally, we rely too much on the conscious mind. If a man suffers from headaches he searches out, with the help of his physician, their cause – discovers whether they come from his eyes, his digestion or his nerves – and purchases the drugs best suited to repair the fault. If he wishes to improve a bad memory, he practices one of the various methods of cognitive training. If he is the victim of a pernicious habit, he's left to counter it by efforts of the will, which too often exhaust his strength, undermine his self-respect, and only lead him deeper into the mire.

How simple in comparison is the method of induced autosuggestion!

He need merely think of the desired end: A head free from pain, a good memory, a mode of life in which his bad habit has no part...and these states are gradually evolved, without him being aware of the operation performed by the subconscious.

But, even so, if each individual difficulty required a fresh treatment – one for the headache, one for the memory, one for the bad habit and so on – then the time needed to practice autosuggestion would form a considerable part of our waking life. Fortunately, Coué has revealed a further simplification. This is obtained by the use of a general formula which sets before the mind the idea of a daily improvement in *every* respect: Mental, physical and moral.

In the original French, this formula runs as follows: "Tous les jours, à tous points de vue, je vais de mieux en mieux." The English translation which Coué considers best is this: "Every day, in every way, I am getting better and better." ("Day by day" can replace "Every day" at the beginning of the phrase if so desired.)

This is a very easy phrase to say: *"Every day, in every way, I'm getting better and better."* The youngest child can understand it, and it possesses a rudimentary rhythm, which exerts a lulling effect on the mind, and so aids in calling up the subconscious.

But this general formula also possesses definite advantages other than mere terseness and convenience. The subconscious, in its character as surveyor over our mental and physical functions, knows far better than the conscious mind the precise failings and weaknesses which have the greatest need of attention. The general formula supplies it with a fund of healing, strengthening power – and leaves it to apply this at the points where the need is most urgent.

It's a matter of common sense that people's ideals of manhood and womanhood vary considerably. For instance, to generalize, the hardened materialist pictures perfection in terms of wealth. The socialite woman wants physical beauty, charm, and the qualities that attract. The sensitive artist is apt to depreciate the powers he possesses and exaggerate those he lacks; while his self-satisfied neighbor can see no good in any virtues but his own.

It's then quite conceivable that a person left free to determine the nature of his autosuggestions, by the light of his conscious desire, might use this power to realize a quality not in itself admirable – or even one that, judged by higher standards, is pernicious. Even supposing that his choice was good, he'd be in danger of over-developing a few characteristics to the detriment of others, and potentially destroy the balance of his personality.

The use of the general formula guards against this. It

saves a man in spite of himself. It avoids the pitfalls into which the conscious mind may lead us by appealing to a more competent authority. Just as we leave the distribution of the food we eat to the subconscious, so may we safely leave our mental food – that of our induced autosuggestions.

The fear that the universal use of this formula could have some sort of a standardizing effect, modifying its users to a uniform pattern, is unfounded. A rigid system of particular suggestions might tend towards such a result, but the general formula leaves every mind free to unfold and develop in the manner most natural to itself. The eternal diversity of our minds can only be increased by the free impulses administered in such a way.

We've seen that the subconscious tide rises to its highest point compatible with conscious thought just before sleep and just after waking, and that the suggestions formulated then are almost assured acceptation. It's these moments that we select for the repetition of the formula.

But before we get into more specifics of the precise method, a word of warning is necessary: Even the most superficial attempt to analyze intellectually a living act is bound to make it appear complex and difficult. So, our consideration of this process has inevitably invested it with a false appearance of difficulty.

*Autosuggestion is, above all things, easy.*

Its greatest enemy is effort. The more simple and unforced the manner of its performance, the more potently and profoundly it works. This is shown by the fact that its most remarkable results have been secured by children and simple French peasants.

It's also here that Coué's directions for the practice differ considerably from those of others. Coué insists upon autosuggestion's easiness, while others tend to complicate it. The latter often leave the impression that autosuggestion is a perplexing business, which only the greatest foresight and supervision can render successful – nothing could be more calculated to throw the beginner off the track, and is exactly the impression Coué wishes to avoid.

We've seen that autosuggestion is a function of the mind, which we spontaneously perform every day of our lives. The more our induced autosuggestions approximate to this spontaneous prototype, the more potent they're likely to be. The fussy attempts of the intellect to dictate the method of processes which lie outside its sphere will only produce conflict, and so condemn our attempt to failure.

Simple directions are amply sufficient, if conscientiously applied, to secure the fullest benefits of which autosuggestion is capable. Before starting it as a daily practice, if you wish, you can take a piece of string and tie in it twenty knots. By this means, you can count with a minimum expenditure of attention, as a devout Catholic counts their prayers on a rosary. The number twenty has no intrinsic virtue; it's merely adopted as a suitable round number.

At night, upon getting into bed, close your eyes, relax

your muscles and take up a comfortable posture. These are no more than the normal actions prior to sleep. Then repeat about twenty times, counting by means of the knots if you like, the general formula: *"Every day, in every way, I'm getting better and better."*

The words should be uttered out loud. That is, loud enough to be audible to your own ears. In this way, the idea is reinforced by the movements of lips and tongue and by the auditory impressions conveyed through the ear. Say it simply, without effort, like a child absently murmuring a nursery rhyme. In this way, you avoid an appeal to the critical faculties of the conscious mind, which would lessen the affect.

When you've gotten used to this exercise, and can say it quite "unconsciously," you can begin to let your voice rise or fall – it doesn't matter which – on *"in every way."* This is perhaps the most important part of the phrase, and therefore can be given a gentle emphasis. But at first don't attempt this accentuation – it will only needlessly complicate things, by requiring more conscious attention (and possible unwanted effort.)

Don't try to think of what you're saying. On the contrary, let the mind wander wherever it will. If it rests on the formula, all the better. If it strays elsewhere, don't worry. As long as your repetition doesn't come to a full-stop, your mind-wandering will be less disturbing than would be the effort to control it.

The sovereign rule is to make no effort, and if this is observed, you'll intuitively fall into the right attitude.

This process of subconscious adaptation may be hastened by a simple suggestion before beginning to repeat the formula. Say to yourself something like, "I'll repeat the formula in such a way as to get its maximum effect." This will help bring about the required conditions much more effectively than any intellectual exercise of thought leading up to induced autosuggestion.

On waking in the morning, repeat the formula in exactly the same manner as when you go to bed at night. Its regular repetition is the foundation stone of the auto-suggestion method, and should never be neglected. In times of happiness and health it may be regarded as an envoy going forth to clear the path of whatever evils may lurk in the future. But we must look on it chiefly as an educator, as a means of leavening the mass of adverse spontaneous suggestions which clog our subconscious, and rob our lives of their true significance.

*"Every day, in every way, I'm getting better and better."*

Say it with faith. When you have said it, your conscious part of the process is completed. Leave the subconscious to do its work undisturbed. Don't be anxious about it, continually scanning yourself for signs of improvement. The farmer doesn't turn over the clods every morning to see if his seed is sprouting. Once sown, it's left till the green blade appears. So it should be with suggestion. Sow the seed, and know the subconscious powers of the mind will bring it to fruition – and all the sooner if your conscious ego is content to let it rest.

Say it with faith! You can only rob induced autosuggestion of its power in one way: By believing that it's powerless. If you believe this, it *becomes* powerless for you. The greater your faith, the more radical and the more rapid will be your results – though if you have only sufficient faith to repeat the phrase twenty times each night and morning, the results will still soon give you the proof you desire, and facts and faith will go on mutually augmenting each other.

# ADDENDUM

*AN ANONYMOUS REPORT
OF COUÉ IN NANCY*

*"One cannot have more than one idea in mind at a time; ideas follow one another without superimposing."*

## MORE EXAMPLES OF COUÉ AT WORK

The old town of Nancy thrills at the mention of Coué. People of every rank and class flock to him, and all are received with an equally benevolent regard, which at once starts many along the way towards recovery. But the deeply touching part to see is, at the close of the session, people who came in bent and gloomy – with an almost hostile feeling caused by pain – go away glad, happy, unconstrained and often radiant with joy, no longer in pain.

Smiling and good natured, with a cheerfulness that's his secret, Mr. Coué holds – so to speak – the hearts of his patients in the hollow of his hand. One by one he addresses the crowd of people who attend his clinic, talking to them as follows:

"Well, Madam, what's your complaint? Oh, you look too much for the *why* and the *where*. What does it matter what causes your pain? You suffer – that is enough. I'll show you how you can get rid of your pain..."

"And you, my dear sir, your varicose sore is improving already. That's fine, that's fine. Do you know you've been here only twice? I congratulate you on having gotten such good results in so short a time. If you continue to make your autosuggestion properly, you'll soon be entirely cured. And you say that you've had this ulcer for ten years? What's the difference? You might've had that sore for twenty years or more, but it'll heal up just the same…"

"And you, you say that you haven't improved at all. Do you know why? Simply because you have no confidence in yourself! When I say that you're better you begin to feel better at once, don't you? Why? Because you *believe in me*. Believe now in yourself, and you'll get just as good results…"

"Oh Madam, not so many details, I beg you! In looking for details you create them, and you would need a list a yard long to hold all your problems. As a matter of fact, it's your *mental outlook* which is wrong. Now, just make up your mind that you're going to get better – and you'll be better very soon. I'm going to show you how to make your autosuggestions. It's as simple and as plain as the Gospel…"

"You say you have an attack of nerves every week. All right. You do as I tell you, and from now on you'll not have them any more…"

"You've been a sufferer from constipation for a long time? What does *the time* matter? You say for forty years. Yes, I heard you. But nonetheless, it's true that you can be cured *tomorrow*. Do you hear? Tomorrow! On condition, of course, that you do just what I tell you to do now, and that you do it just as I show you…"

"Ah, you suffer from glaucoma, Madam. I can't

absolutely promise a complete cure of that. I'm not quite sure. But that doesn't mean that a cure is impossible. For I've seen a lady from Chalon-sur-Saône and another one from Toul cured…"

"Well, Mademoiselle, as you've not had any nervous attacks since the last time you came here, and before that you used to have them every day, you're cured. Nonetheless, come and see me once in a while so that I may keep you moving along in the right direction…"

"Your feeling of oppression will vanish just as soon as your lesions have disappeared and when you assimilate your food properly. That will all come about in good time, but don't put the cart before the horse. It's the same with oppression as with heart trouble, both generally disappear pretty quickly…"

Speaking to a child (in a clear and commanding voice): "Shut your eyes. I won't talk to you about lesions or anything like that. You wouldn't understand it, anyway. The pain in your chest is going and you don't feel like coughing anymore…"

To one who complains of fatigue: "Well, I have the same complaint. There are days when I, too, am tired of receiving people. Nonetheless, I receive them all day long. Don't say *'I can't help it.'* One can always rise above one's self…" (The idea of being tired brings about that languid feeling of fatigue, while the idea of having a duty to perform always gives us the necessary strength to do it.)

"Whatever may be the cause that prevents your walking, it's going to disappear – bit by bit, every day. You know the old proverb: *Heaven helps those who help themselves.* Stand up for a little while, several times each day, supporting yourself between two people. Don't say to yourself 'My kidneys are too weak, I can't do it.' But say out loud, and with a firm voice: *'I can, I can, I can...'*"

"After you've repeated *'Every day, in every way, I'm getting better and better,'* you add: 'The persons that have been following me do not follow me now, they *cannot* follow me anymore...'"

"What I've been telling you is very true: It's enough for you *to think* that you have no more pain for the pain to disappear. Therefore, please don't think that it might come again, for it then will surely come back..." (A woman murmurs "What *patience* he has, what a wonderfully painstaking man!")

"Whatever *we think* comes true for us. We must therefore not think anything detrimental to ourselves..."

"Ah! *To will* and *to desire* is not the same thing..."

"To become stronger as you become older may seem to be paradoxical, but it's true..."

"This obsession of yours appears to be something of a real nightmare. Know the people you detested are now becoming friends: You're going to like them and they will like you..."

"You, my dear sir, are in pain. But I tell you that from this day on that which causes the pain is going to disappear. No matter whether it's called 'arthritis,' or whether it goes by any other name, your subconscious will do the thing needful to banish the cause. And as the cause is being removed, little by little, the pain also will vanish and in a short time there will be nothing left of it but the memory…"

"Your stomach doesn't function properly, it's more or less distended. Well, as I told you just now: Your digestive organs are going to start to work better and better. The distention of your stomach is also going to disappear gradually. As your entire system regains force and elasticity, your stomach will therefore benefit, and slowly get back into proper form to carry out more and more easily the movements necessary to pass the nourishment it contains into the intestines. At the same time, the pouch formed by the enlarged stomach will diminish in size, the food will no longer stagnate in that pouch, and consequently will disappear…"

"To you, Mademoiselle, I say that whatever lesions you may have in your liver, your body is doing whatever is necessary to cause those lesions to heal up, more and more every day. By degrees, the symptoms from which you now suffer will lessen and finally disappear entirely. Your liver is going to function more and more in a normal way, secreting an alkaline bile which is no longer acidulous but right in quantity and quality so that it will pass into the intestinal tract in proper condition and aid intestinal digestion…"

"My child, you just listen: Every time you feel another attack coming on, you'll hear my voice saying to you with lightning-like rapidity, *'No, no my friend you're not going to have that attack!'* It will be gone before it really comes…"

"I've told you, and I repeat my dear sir, that your varicose sore is going to heal. From this day on, interlacing granulations will form at the bottom of your ulcer, and growing they'll gradually fill the hole now existing. At the same time, the ledges will reapproach each other in every direction, both in height and width, until they touch and heal up altogether…"

"You have a rupture, you say. Well, it can and it will be cured. Your subconscious self will act in such a way that the rupture which exists in your peritoneum is going to heal up by degrees. The hole will get smaller and smaller every day, until it's completely closed and you have no rupture anymore…"

"And you, my dear sir, who have glaucoma or some sort of cataract: I tell you that from this day on the lesions which you have in your eyes will begin to heal up. And as they do so, by degrees you'll notice that your eyes are getting better and better, and you'll be able to see farther and much more clearly…"

"You say you have eczema. This affection will disappear rapidly. I said *rapidly*, you understand? The cause which brought about this affection is going to vanish. And naturally, the cause being removed, the symptoms will likewise vanish. If there's stinging or itching in the affected parts, you'll notice that it lessens day by day. If there's a slight discharge, it also will be less and less every day. In short, as your skin peels off in the form of scales, you'll find it replaced by a new elastic skin of natural color…"

"The intestinal inflammation will diminish gradually, and the blood which sometimes accompanies your stools will at the same time become less frequent until it stops altogether, and you'll be cured…"

Anemia: "Your blood is becoming more and more rich and abundant, until it has improved to the natural state of a healthy person. In this way, your anemia and all the annoying conditions that follow in its train will have entirely vanished…"

"Every time you begin to have pains, say right away: *'It passes, it passes.'* Say it quickly, rapidly – like a firing barrage. You must learn how to *use* autosuggestion, and after having had a few lessons, you'll not need me anymore unless you *think* that you need me…"

"The experiments have been very successful. If you don't get any sleep, it's because you're making efforts. It's enough to say *'I am going to sleep, I am going to sleep'* – humming it like the sound of a flying bee. If this proves unsuccessful it's simply because you're not doing it right…"

"All that is periodical is self-acquired. From childhood, they've heard it said that Aunt Gertrude has it, Cousin Mary has it, etc. – and they *assume* that they too are going to have it…"

"To say 'Provided I don't have neuralgia' is as much as saying *that you expect to have it*. Don't give a thought to an ailment of any kind – otherwise that which you expect and are afraid of is going to happen…"

"You're constipated because you *think* you are. Just *think the contrary* and the contrary will happen…"

"These fears and aversions must disappear. You have in yourself the instrument of your recovery. Drive them away, let them drop like crumbs from your table. Nobody in the world can exercise any influence on you unless you *permit* it. Don't come next time to tell me that you're not better – *you will be better*. And don't use willpower. Don't even use the words 'I will' – I forbid you, if there's anything at all to forbid…"

"If you have a broken bone go to the hospital immediately. Suggestion does not reset or repair broken bones, but directs and controls the organs, muscles, nerves, etc.…"

Coué: "Do you follow your diet for albumen?"
Patient: "I don't like the milk food."
Coué: "Well, imagine that you *do* like it…"

"As regards to these itchings, you've been here three times. Impress the thought on your mind *that they will never come back again*. If you're afraid that they're going to occur again, they surely will. Even after you've improved, continue to see me from time to time, in order that I may encourage you to keep yourself in the right direction..."

Patient: "One may force one's self to think, doctor?"
Coué: "No need to *force* yourself to practice the method – that comes quite naturally. It's the same for me, you know..."

Patient: "I cannot say 'I cannot' when I think 'I can.'"
Coué: "Do as I tell you. It's I who gives you a lesson, not you to me..."

Bronchitis: "You have bronchitis and are taking the Valda tablets. That's all right to calm irritation. Suggestion will make *the cause* of irritation disappear..."

"You've seen your doctor about it, follow the diet he's prescribed for you. Madam, you *must* follow the treatment prescribed by your doctor. And make suggestions at the same time. The one doesn't prevent or prohibit the other. On the contrary, *I too prescribe for you...*"

"There's no healer here, but a gentleman who teaches you what to do to heal yourself..."

Neuralgia: "Whatever the cause may be for your headaches, your body will do all that's necessary to make that cause disappear, gradually. And, of course, in the same measure: As the cause disappears, your neuralgia will be less frequent and less violent – until in the near future it will have vanished altogether. You feel, by the way, every time that I pass my hand across your forehead, it takes away some of the pain, and in a moment – when you open your eyes – you'll find that you're currently entirely free from it..."

Patient: "I suffocate, especially in hot weather."
Coué: "You've seen your doctor?"
Patient: "I've seen six doctors. They said it's nervousness, but they did nothing for it."
Coué: "Yes, it's nervousness, but we're going to help *you* to get rid of it..."

Upon conclusion of working with everyone: "You've heard the advice I've just given you. Well, in order to transform my suggestions into realities, here's what you must do: As long as you live, every morning before rising and every evening as soon as you're in bed, close your eyes. Then repeat, twenty times with your lips moving – which is essential – and counting mechanically on a string with twenty knots in it, the following phrase: *'Every day, in every way, I am getting better and better.'*

"Don't think of anything in particular, as the words *'in every way'* apply to everything. Make this autosuggestion with confidence, with faith – with the certainty that you're going to obtain what you desire. The greater the faith of the patient, the greater and the more rapid the results will be.

"Moreover, if at any time during the day or night you feel any physical or mental discomfort, say to yourself that you'll not consciously contribute toward it – *but that you're going to compel it to disappear.*

"Then isolate yourself as much as possible and pass your hand across your forehead if it's something mental – or over the painful body part if it's something physical – and repeat with extreme rapidity, moving the lips: *'It passes, it passes, it passes,'* for as long as necessary. With a little practice, the mental or physical discomfort will disappear in twenty to twenty-five seconds. Repeat again whenever necessary.

"In this, as well as in other autosuggestions, it's necessary to act with confidence, faith – and above all, *without effort.*

"If formerly you've been in the habit of subconsciously making bad autosuggestions to yourself, now knowing what I've taught, you must not let those bad subconscious autosuggestions occur again. And, if in spite of all I've instructed, you still persist in making them, then you have only yourselves to blame and better strike your breast and say: 'Mea culpa, mea culpa, mea maxima culpa.'"

Now, if a grateful admirer of the work – and of its founder – may be permitted to say a few closing words. Since Mr. Coué tells us that it's the imagination which makes us act, and that this is the basis of his method, I would like to add: *The pillars of his structure are the thousands of cures obtained.*

And the crowning part – the most magnificent crowning part – is his noble admission the power is *in you*. In each of us is this power. This constitutes not only an immense benefit for suffering humanity, but also is a tribute to its creator. Each of us can adapt this method to our own personal creed. And for all – whether religious believers, skeptics or free-thinkers – Coué's method teaches us how to deliver ourselves from mental or physical pain that's unjustified, by use of the simple yet marvelous process: *It passes!*

As for those who reject this method, ignorant of the secret of its force, I'll ask you one question: Do you also reject the lightbulb because you don't know the secret of the power of electricity? You don't know – you *can't* know – what this blessed method can do, and will do, to restore you mentally and physically. But in *living and practicing it*, you will know. It's sure to help you gain victory in the mastery of yourself.

*EVERY DAY, IN EVERY WAY, I'M GETTING BETTER AND BETTER...*

For More Information Visit:

*www.radicalcounselor.com*

Made in the USA
Las Vegas, NV
27 July 2023

75323014R00080